The
Family
Handbook of
Hospice Care

Fairview Hospice, Fairview Health Services

Fairview Press
Minneapolis

Published by Fairview Press, 2450 Riverside Avenue, Minneapolis, MN 55454. Fairview Press is a division of Fairview Health Services, a community-focused health system, affiliated with the University of Minnesota, providing a complete range of services, from the prevention of illness and injury to care for the most complex medical conditions. For a free current catalog of Fairview Press titles, call toll-free 1-800-544-8207, or visit our Web site at www.fairviewpress.org.

ISBN-10: 1-57749-090-8
ISBN-13: 978-1-57749-090-6
Library of Congress Cataloging-in-Publication Data
The family handbook of hospice care / Fairview Hospice, Fairview Health Services
     p.   cm.
   Includes bibliographical references and index.
   ISBN 1-57749-090-8 (pbk. : alk. paper)
   1. Hospice care. I. Fairview Hospice. II. Fairview Health Services.
R726.8F354 1999
362.1'756--dc21   99-042786
                   CIP
First Printing: October 1999; Revised: January 2008
Printed in the United States of America

Writer: Kären Hess, Innovative Programming Systems Inc.
Cover: Laurie Ingram
Interior: Percolator Graphic Design

Medical Disclaimer:
This publication is designed to provide accurate and authoritative information in regard to the subject matter covered. It is sold with the understanding that the publisher is not engaged in the provision or practice of medical, nursing, or professional healthcare advice or services in any jurisdiction. If medical advice or other ?professional assistance is required, the services of a qualified and competent professional should be sought. Fairview Press is not responsible or liable, directly or indirectly, for any form of damages whatsoever resulting from the use (or misuse) of information contained in or implied by these documents.

Other things may change us,
but we start and end with family.
—Anthony Brandt

With deep gratitude, we dedicate this book to the patients and families whom we have been privileged to know and serve over the years. You have inspired us. May the blessings you have given others through your love and service come back to you.

Acknowledgments

Families and caregivers have often asked Fairview Hospice for written information to help them care for their terminally ill loved ones at home. *The Family Handbook of Hospice Care* has been a dream of Fairview Hospice staff for many years. This dream became a reality when Fairview Press recognized the value of the project and offered to assist us. We wish to thank the following people whose contributions were particularly helpful in the preparation of this book.

Our hospice patients and families inspire us daily to learn new and better ways of supporting them as they journey together into an uncertain future. We would especially like to thank Katherine Baumgartner, whose beloved father, Olaf Kaasa, was a patient of Fairview Hospice. Her perspective as a family caregiver was extremely valuable in creating this book.

Our Fairview Hospice staff, who conceived the very idea for this book, gave unselfishly of their time to convey the essence of our message to the writer. We would especially like to thank the core committee members for their many hours discussing and editing the text under tight deadlines. These individuals include Kathleen Lucas, Virginia Bender, Tami Schoenbauer, Steve Sims, Jean Campbell, and Mary Hagen.

Our writer, Kären Hess, listened intently, revised repeatedly without ego, and captured the essence of the message beautifully. Her openness, willingness to learn, and easygoing style made this book possible.

The Family Handbook of Hospice Care would continue to be a loose collection of miscellaneous booklets and photocopied handouts if Marne Oberg and Lyndsay Hall of Fairview Public Relations had not recognized its potential and called Fairview Press to explore the feasibility of writing a book.

The generous contributions of two other individuals have helped turn this book into an excellent resource for patients and families. Larry Beresford, a former senior writer for the National Hospice and Palliative Care Organization, took time out from his very busy schedule to write a thought-provoking foreward, and Kristin Dungan of Fairview's legal department was kind enough to act as a consultant for the legal sections.

To the staff at Fairview Press, a very special thank you for providing the talent and expertise necessary to deliver a wonderful resource for hospice families and staff everywhere. Lane Stiles understood our dream and saw the possibilities. Stephanie Billecke, our editor, also deserves enormous gratitude. She was our shepherd and coach, possessed of a great sense of commitment, dedication, humor, and patience. Without Stephanie, we would still be dreaming.

CONTENTS

Foreword

The basic message of this book—and of the hospice approach of compassionate care for the dying—is twofold: "Caregiving may be the hardest thing you will ever do," the authors state. "Even so, most people who have done it say the challenge is worthwhile."

For three decades, highly motivated hospice professionals and volunteers throughout this country have striven mightily to make the final chapter of life less painful, less difficult, more manageable, and, at its best, more meaningful for both patients and their families. Yet too often hospice is dimly understood, misunderstood, feared, or avoided.

When hospice enters your life, in all likelihood it means your loved one is seriously ill and likely will not survive his or her illness. Despite people's instinctive fears, hospice won't make a loved one's death come any sooner or with greater certainty. Hospice is all about making the very best of this frightening situation, helping you to play the hand you have been dealt so that years later you will feel you did the right thing for your loved one. But before you can allow hospice's support into your life, you must begin to confront the painful reality of an impending death.

In the spring of 1999, public opinion research conducted for the National Hospice Foundation of Arlington, Virginia, showed that while Americans have a vague notion of what hospice care is, few understand how it works or that Medicare pays for it. Few are aware that hospice provides emotional support and pain relief, and only 13 percent say they would call their local hospice if a family member or close friend were confronting a terminal illness.

Yet, in recent years, deeply held fears about how Americans expect to be treated by the conventional healthcare system at the end of life have been widely documented. The 1997 focus group study, "The Quest to Die with Dignity," issued by a national coalition of citizen health advocacy groups called American Health Decisions, concluded that Americans of all ages and races fear a medically intrusive, mechanical pathway to death. Yet they avoid doing the one thing that could make the greatest difference—discussing their fears and wishes with their family or doctor. In fact, the National Hospice Foundation discovered that Americans are more willing to talk about safe sex or drug abuse with their children than to discuss end-of-life care with an aging parent.

Hospices from coast to coast report that many patients are referred to hospice care very late in their illness—often days or even hours before death. That makes it difficult for hospice to offer much more than short-term crisis management, though a peaceful, comfortable, self-determined final chapter might have been possible. A comfortable end may afford priceless opportunities to say meaningful farewells, to heal long-standing emotional rifts, and to find an element of closure in relationships.

Over and over, family survivors say, "If only we'd known about hospice sooner." Perhaps for some family caregivers, this book will forestall that complaint. Hospice can't change the sad ending of these all-too-common human dramas, but it may be able to make them more tolerable. Ultimately, however, as the authors note, "There is never enough time for all that we want to say or do. It is never really 'okay' for someone to die. Don't expect to accept it right away"—despite what you may have heard about Elisabeth Kübler-Ross's five stages of dying.

The Family Handbook of Hospice Care is written for family caregivers of patients with life-threatening illnesses, and for good reason. Often a patient's nearest family member, typically a spouse or adult child, is thrust into the role of decision maker. This caregiver plays a central part in managing the patient's care, if the patient is to live at home throughout the illness. And because the caregiver may long outlive the patient, he or she will want to look back on the experience knowing that the best possible caregiving decisions were made.

The authors address the many fears and uncertainties about terminal illness, hospice, and caregiving in clear, simple terms. They illustrate the caregiving process through brief vignettes tracing a hypothetical hospice patient and spouse, John and Ella, from their initial fears about hospice through Ella's grieving process a year after John's death. The book also contains helpful checklists, brief inspirational quotes, and references to other caregiving texts.

This book doesn't sugarcoat the immensely challenging realities of caring for a terminally ill loved one. It covers such key issues as the multitude of negative feelings that can arise, the physical challenges of skin and mouth care, and the nitty-gritty details of constipation, diarrhea, and incontinence. It focuses on the centrality of pain management and pain medications in the hospice process. It offers suggestions for an effective diet—as well as for dealing with the emotions that often arise when the patient stops eating and drinking. The authors offer helpful hints on fundamental legal and financial issues, as well as on the powerful and unavoidable reality of grief.

Among the many practical discussions in the book are the cornerstones of the hospice approach and the four key considerations for preparing areas in the home for caregiving: accessibility, safety, convenience, and cleanliness. The authors recommend keeping a written daily care log to track hospice team members, care needs, essential household tasks, and pain reports. But amid the many practical aspects of caregiving, the authors never let the reader forget that a terminal illness has tremendous spiritual implications as well—regardless of the patient's and family's religious beliefs—and that there is still a place for hope.

Finally, to help demystify the physical changes that accompany the final transition, the authors discuss some of the signs of approaching death—right up to the very moment of death. "A moment—that's how long it takes for your loved one to leave his or her physical body," they observe. And for family caregivers everywhere, they offer this benediction:

> *Death is the conclusion of the journey you have made with your loved one to his or her final rest. It will be sad. It will hurt. But it should also be comforting to know that you and your loved one have successfully completed the journey together.*

Larry Beresford is a freelance healthcare journalist in Oakland, California, a frequent contributor to the publications of the National Hospice and Palliative Care Organization, Alexandria, Virginia, and the author of *The Hospice Handbook* (Boston: Little, Brown & Co., 1993).

You're Not Alone: How Hospice Can Help

*You matter because you are you. You matter to the
last moment of your life, and we will do all we can,
not only to help you die peacefully, but to live until
you die.*

—Dr. Cicely Saunders, founder of the first hospice

*It was 4 a.m. and Ella had helped her frail husband, John, to his bed-
side commode. He had terminal cancer and was no longer able to
make it to the bathroom, even with a walker. He had fallen off the
commode and was now writhing in pain. She did not dare try to move
him. Frantic, she called 911. An ambulance arrived, and paramedics
skillfully lifted him onto a stretcher and wheeled him to the ambulance. As they drove away, Ella began sobbing. Although she desper-
ately wanted to continue caring for her husband of forty-nine years at
home, she knew she was no longer up to the task. She called her son,
Tim, and asked him to come take her to the hospital. When they
arrived at the emergency room, a young doctor greeted them. After
introducing herself, the doctor told them they could take John home.
No bones were broken, and his pain was under control. There was
nothing more the hospital could do for him. But John and Ella did
have some options. She handed Ella a small pamphlet called "How
Hospice Can Help" and said she'd like to have a hospice staff member
stop by in the morning to talk to John and her.*

Ella was stunned. She couldn't send John to a hospice. She could not bear the thought. But the next morning, the hospice nurse put Ella's and John's fears to rest as she explained how hospice could not only allow John to stay at home, but also help Ella continue to care for him. Hospice was the answer for this loving couple.

WHAT IS HOSPICE?

The great events of life, as we observe them, are still clearly recognizable as journeys.... Out of centuries of experience has come the repeated observation that death appears to be a process rather than an event, a form of passage for human life.

—Sandol Stoddard, *The Hospice Movement: A Better Way of Caring for the Dying*

Hospice is a philosophy of care for the terminally ill. It refers to the steadily growing concept of humane, compassionate care in a variety of settings. Hospice care can be provided in the patient's home or apartment, an assisted living facility, a nursing home, an inpatient hospice facility, or a special wing in a hospital. Ideally, the care is provided in the patient's home or in a homelike setting. If your loved one will receive hospice care in a nursing home, or a long-term care facility, see page 124.

Although the setting may vary, hospice provides physical, emotional, and spiritual support to those who are dying and to their family and caregivers. Its goal is to make death as painless and meaningful as possible. It is a special way of caring that offers help and hope to the patient and family members. Hospice focuses not on dying, but on living well and with dignity during the time that is left. Hospice also offers grief and bereavement services for survivors of the patient.

Hospice views life as a journey. Its goal is to help people complete life's journey with hope, comfort, dignity, and companionship. Hospice care is rooted in the centuries-old tradition of preparing gifts for those embarking on a long journey. Hospice seeks to help the terminally ill patient experience the richness of life each step of the way. Implicit in hospice care is the message, "I will journey with you. Although I cannot go through the door at the end of the journey, I can be with you to the threshold."

The word *hospice* goes back to medieval times. It described a place of shelter and rest for weary and ill travelers returning from religious pilgrimages. It later came to refer to a place where wounded crusaders could rest and have their injuries treated. Later yet, it referred to a house of rest for pilgrims, travelers, the destitute, and the sick. Our words *hospital* and *hospitality* come from the word hospice.

Dr. Cicely Saunders began the modern hospice movement in 1967. She established St. Christopher's Hospice near London and was the medical director from its founding in 1967 until 1985. Its purpose was to provide pain and symptom control together with compassionate care. Fittingly, this first hospice was named after the patron saint of travelers. Dr. Saunders viewed her hospice as a stopping place for weary travelers who were nearing the end of their earthly pilgrimage.

The first hospice in the United States was the Connecticut Hospice, Inc., founded in 1974. Unlike its English counterpart, this hospice focused on providing in-home services. The National Hospice Organization (NHO) was formed in 1978 in Washington, D.C. The planners hoped that 400 people would attend the first meeting; however, over 1,000 came. Today, now known as the National Hospice and Palliative Care Organization (NHPCO), it is the largest nonprofit representing hospice care professionals in the United States. Currently the United States has over 3,000 hospice programs.

Dying at Home

Dying invariably creates a wider awareness of life.
—Daniel Tobin, M.D., *Peaceful Dying*

Many years ago, people died at home. Death was viewed as natural, and family members witnessed it firsthand. With medical advances, however, it became common for people to spend their last days in a hospital, at times alone. The focus of hospital physicians and nurses was (and is) on finding a cure or, at least, prolonging life. However, a nationwide Gallup survey conducted for NHPCO found that nine out of ten Americans say they would prefer to be cared for and die at home.

We are beginning to come full circle. More and more people are choosing to die at home, and they are taking advantage of the supportive resources of hospice. Although it brings great sadness, caring for a terminally ill loved one until the end of life is a major accomplishment. Countless hospice patients and families know that living when one's days are numbered can be a time of deepening relationships, spiritual growth, healing, and peace. During the dying process, the truths that underlie life can emerge with irrefutable clarity.

Although hospice provides care for the dying, it stresses the positive aspects of living each day as fully as possible, as comfortably as possible, with the support of loved ones and a highly trained hospice care team. Hospice helps people make the best of today when the tomorrows are limited.

THE CORNERSTONES OF HOSPICE

Hospice rests squarely on four cornerstones:
1. The family as the primary caregiver.
2. The support of a well-educated hospice care team.
3. Comfort care and the control of pain.
4. Living life with hope in the face of death.

The Family as the Primary Caregiver

In hospice, the family no longer sits by helplessly, watching a loved one die a slow and painful death. They no longer cling to false hope for a miracle cure. Instead, they help their loved one through the process of dying and prepare themselves for the forthcoming loss. Whoever constitutes the patient's family, whether a close companion or friends and relatives, they can actively participate in meeting their loved one's needs and fulfilling his or her wishes when possible.

The Hospice Care Team

The hospice care team includes members from many professions. A nurse is always on call. The attending physician (usually the patient's primary or family doctor) and hospice medical director oversee the care plan. A hospice nurse coordinates the care plan and provides specialized palliative (pain relieving) services. A home health aide can assist with personal care and light house-keeping. A social worker can be there to listen and offer emotional support, counseling, and referrals to community support services. A hospice spiritual care provider, also called a chaplain, (or a member of the clergy, depending on individual preference) may provide spiritual care. The team may include a variety of therapists, including physical, occupational, respiratory, nutritional, speech, massage, and music therapists. It may also include a pharmacist. A bereavement coordinator is available to support the family after their loved one's death. The hospice team is there to offer support while respecting the family's needs, beliefs, and values.

Trained volunteers also provide a variety of services. They can listen and offer emotional support, run errands, do light house-keeping, help prepare meals, act as companions, and provide short-term respite care to give the family caregiver a break. The hospital experience is supplemented and often replaced by an end-of-life care team that not only believes in the uniqueness of each person, but will help the patient find his or her own way of dying.

Comfort Care and Control of Pain

Hospice neither prolongs life nor hastens death. It emphasizes patient comfort through the effective management of pain and other symptoms. The hospice nurse and team members are trained in comfort care, which may include medication and therapy.

A Focus on Living and Hope

> In the hospice setting, you ask: How does someone have hope? How do you give meaning to life? Hope gets redefined; it becomes a day without pain or discomfort, living seven months instead of six, or being filled with gratitude for the little things.
>
> —Dale Swan, hospice spiritual care provider

Once pain is under control, patients can focus on living, and most will come to accept death as a reality. In our society, death is often viewed as an enemy and we hesitate to talk about death. Some people, when informed of their terminal illness, die emotionally— they give up all hope. Hospice seeks to keep hope alive even though it is no longer realistic to hope for a cure.

The hospice patient can hope for many things: to see a son or daughter's upcoming wedding or graduation, to get out in the sun, to see the seasons change, to see old friends again, to heal family rifts, to attend to financial matters, to say goodbye.

Hospice views the dying process as a gradual "letting go" rather than "giving up hope." The focus is on living and turning the remaining time into quality time. To reduce the distress of dying, hospice provides human warmth and concern as well as medical expertise. For many people, intimacy with death increases their potential to discover the meaning of life.

WHO MIGHT BENEFIT FROM HOSPICE?

Hospice is reserved for individuals who are terminally ill and whose life expectancy is measured in weeks or months rather than years. (Generally, the person has six months or fewer to live.) Although many patients are referred to hospice by their physician, patients and their families may contact hospice directly.

Hospice care is appropriate when an individual's illness no longer responds to curative treatment. Hospice care is important to AIDS patients, patients with end-stage congestive heart failure or lung disease, patients with end-stage cancer, patients with advanced Alzheimer's or Parkinson's disease or ALS, pediatric patients with certain congenital disorders, and anyone for whom hope of a cure is gone. When patients have run out of treatment options, or when they no longer want to undergo painful or unpleasant treatments, hospice offers hope. With hospice, the focus shifts from curing the disease to caring for the person.

Unfortunately, many patients are referred to hospice quite late in their illness. Hospice professionals have found that patients who enroll early have more time to build trusting relationships with their hospice care team. Early enrollment also helps the hospice team get pain and other symptoms under control—and can often prevent these symptoms altogether. The sooner patients enroll in hospice, the more likely they are to benefit from the comfort and support that hospice has to offer.

MAKING THE DECISION

Hospice offers many benefits for the patient and his or her family, including the following:

- Hospice addresses the physical, social, emotional, and spiritual needs of the dying person and the family.

- Comfort, dignity, and quality of life are the priorities.

- Hospice nurses are on call twenty-four hours a day, seven days a week.

- Hospice offers caregiver support.

- Living at home with hospice support helps the patient and his or her family members maintain a sense of normalcy in their lives.

- Hospice team members are specially trained in working with terminally ill people and their families and are experts in pain control and symptom relief.

- The patient and family members have more time to prepare for the loved one's death.

- Hospice can place the patient in an inpatient setting when necessary to improve symptom control or to give caregivers a break from their responsibilities.

- Hospice provides grief support for the survivors.

Once patient and family decide that hospice is the right choice, it is important that both the patient and the family members understand their roles.

THE ROLE OF THE PATIENT

When an illness is diagnosed as life threatening or incurable, it is sad and frightening. However, in one sense it may be a blessing, because the patient and the family have been given the gift of knowing they have limited, precious time.

Patients are kept informed about their condition and treatment alternatives, and they are asked to participate in formulating the care plan. After a plan is established, the patient must do his or her part. This includes following the nutritional portion of the plan and faithfully taking pain medications as prescribed. It is important to keep pain under control rather than try to reduce it after it occurs.

Patients are asked to be honest about how they feel and what they would like to do. If they want a quiet afternoon alone, they need to say so. If they are concerned about being a burden, about financial matters, or have a fear of loss, especially of their independence, these issues need to be discussed.

THE ROLE OF THE FAMILY

Although caring for a dying loved one can be stressful, it gives families the chance to be close to their loved one at the end of his or her life. The family has a number of responsibilities. First, to provide a safe, comfortable environment. Second, to keep the hospice team informed of any problems or changes in the patient or the care plan. Third, to be there for their loved one—to give support, to talk through issues, and to share their loved one's journey. Fourth, to assist with their loved one's personal care, attending to eating, hygiene, position, comfort, and other needs. (The hospice team will teach the family the necessary skills.) Finally, to attend to errands, meals, medications, financial applications, and other practical matters.

Routine daily caregiving is not covered by Medicare or insurance plans, except during extreme crisis periods. It is usually performed by family members, with help from friends. In long-term care facilities, caregiving is performed by facility staff.

Usually, one family member is the primary caregiver. Sometimes two or more family members share this responsibility. In other instances, the primary caregiver may not be a family member, but someone who is very close to the patient, such as a friend.

The entire family, as well as close friends, must work together to surround the patient with love and to help each other "let go." Everyone involved, including the patient, should be preparing for the inevitable.

How each family comes together will be different. Some families are very close, both emotionally and geographically. Such families are likely to work well together in support of their loved one. Other families may have strained relationships or be separated by distance. It will be more difficult for these families. In some cases, one or two family members may be relied on—and one or two family members may never come through. No matter what the family situation, the primary caregiver is not alone. The hospice team is there to help.

THE ROLE OF HOSPICE

Hospice offers a wide variety of well-coordinated services to provide for the patient's physical, emotional, and spiritual needs. In addition to the support team of physicians, nurses, home health aides, social workers, spiritual care providers, therapists, and volunteers, families may request the help of other professionals such as bankers, lawyers, funeral directors, and the like. The hospice team will help arrange these meetings.

A member of the hospice team can teach family members specific caregiving techniques such as turning, positioning, transferring, bathing, and giving medications. Another team member may arrange for a wheelchair, walker, bedside commode, hospital bed, oxygen, and other equipment as needed. Team members can also provide information about grief support groups and other resources. Volunteers might offer respite care to give family members or the caregiver a break. The specific services will vary depending upon patient and family needs.

THE CARE PLAN

The care plan is a vital part of hospice. It addresses all the medical, nursing, and other care required and determines who will carry out each portion of the plan. It includes not only the physical needs of the patient, but the emotional and spiritual needs of patient and family as well. An effective care plan must begin and end with the patient and family. To be effective the patient and family must be involved so that the plan is designed to meet the patient's needs.

Tears and Smiles:
Coping with a Terminal Illness

*The perception that "nothing more can be done"
has often had a devastating effect on both patients
and families. But even though the disease may be
incurable, much more can be done to ease the pain
and suffering of the patient and at the same time
involve family members in the patient's care.*

—The National Hospice Organization, *Meeting the
Challenge for a Special Kind of Caring*

*3 a.m. John tossed restlessly in bed, countless fears causing sleepless-
ness. Since beginning hospice care, he was thankful, yet apprehensive.
How would his illness affect the household and those he loved? Could
Ella cope with the burden of caring for him? How would his children
react? Did he want his friends to see him in this condition? Would he
suffer? Would he be prepared? As he reached for the glass of water by
his bedside, Ella roused and asked, "Darling, are you all right? Are
you in pain? Do you need to talk?"*

*John heard the love in his wife's voice, felt the gentle touch of her
hand on his arm, and responded, "No, Sweetheart, I'm not in pain.
I'm just worried about how we are going to handle this dying business. I don't want to be a burden to you or the kids."*

*"Nonsense," Ella replied. "We love you and love helping you with
this. We need to do this for you and for ourselves. Besides, we have our*

fiftieth wedding anniversary coming up next month. We'd better start making some plans in the morning, okay?"

"Okay," John murmured as his thoughts turned to their long marriage and upcoming golden anniversary. He soon drifted off to sleep reassured by the presence of her love.

According to a Harris Poll, 96 percent of Americans said they would want to be told if they had cancer, and 85 percent would want a realistic estimate of how long they had to live. Yet, when patients and families are told, "There is nothing more we can do," it can be shattering. While this statement is really not true, it is said all the time. According to hospice philosophy, much can be done. Hospice care affirms life—it allows people to live until they die, sharing the end of their life with people important to them.

Patients are likely to feel anxious, fearful, and depressed. They are losing control in their lives, their self-image is changing, and they fear potential pain and suffering. Perhaps most distressing is their fear of the unknown.

Likewise, family members face their own anxieties and fears because of their loved one's suffering—and because nothing they do will change the fact that their loved one is going to die. They sometimes resent the responsibilities thrust upon them, and they may feel guilty because of this resentment.

As a caregiver, you may think your feelings are crazy, selfish, or unreasonable. The fact is, your feelings are valid expressions of your inner emotions. They must be acknowledged, no matter how strange or unreasonable they may seem to you.

The emotions surrounding death and dying have been studied for centuries. Many books are available to help you understand this universal human experience; however, each person's death is unique. As you read about the physical and emotional realities of death and dying, take what helps and ignore what doesn't.

THE STAGES OF DYING—IN THEORY

A quarter century ago, Dr. Elisabeth Kübler-Ross wrote the classic book, *On Death and Dying*, which identified five stages of dying that a terminally ill patient goes through: denial and isolation, anger, bargaining, depression, and acceptance. Although these stages are frequently cited in books about the dying experience, they are only a theory. Your loved one may experience one or more of these stages (not necessarily in the order presented), and she may go back and forth between the stages throughout the dying process.

Denial and Isolation

*Denial is not necessarily negative. There is a fine
line between denial and hope.*

—Jean Campbell, hospice social worker

In *denial and isolation* the patient refuses to accept the inevitability of their own death: "No, this can't be happening to me. This happens to other people, not me." A patient in denial will usually refuse to talk about it, perhaps believing that not talking about it will make it go away. Such patients often seek out second, third, and even fourth medical opinions. During this stage the patient may experience shock. "Why now? I've just retired!" "But I've always taken such good care of myself."

Denial is a powerful tool to help us adapt to a painful reality. In the short run, denial allows us to adjust to bad news until we can mobilize all other defenses. Ongoing denial, however, can be debilitating. It's as if you're saying, "I can't deal with this, so I'm going to act like it's not happening."

Unfortunately, some patients get stuck in this stage of disbelief, refusing to face the reality needed to move on to a peaceful death. They may refuse consolation and die in isolation, tense and fearful.

Family members also experience denial, refusing to accept the inevitable. They may also experience shock. News of a loved one's terminal illness violates their view of how the world is supposed to be. "How can this happen when we're expecting our first grandchild?" "It's not fair. The doctors are wrong." In such cases, relationships may not be strengthened, important financial matters may go unattended, and intense feelings of guilt may follow the loved one's death.

Although denial can sometimes create communication barriers, it can also help the patient move from one stage of dying to the next.

Anger

> *It's perfectly natural to feel anger when you're supporting the dying process of someone you love. Let the anger out. The universe can absorb it. Our bodies can't. … Freeing it—accepting and expressing it—helps you and the dying person prepare for your loss and can help you both move toward acceptance.*
>
> —**Deborah Duda**, *Coming Home*

Anger is another stage in the dying process. Once the reality of the situation sinks in, patients may experience anger, even rage. "Why me?" Family members and medical staff may bear the brunt of this anger. "I told you I was sick. Why didn't you listen to me?" "My doctor is incompetent." "The lab fouled up." Along with these emotions come envy and resentment. "I've lived a good life. Why not strike down those who have nothing to contribute to the world?" "Why didn't I have better doctors?" "How can God let this happen to me?"

Family members often feel angry too. They may resent that their loved one didn't take better care of himself or herself. They may feel cheated, now that their time with their loved one is coming to a premature close. "How can she leave me like this?" They want their old world back. They may even resent the demands now being made on their time and energy. Unfortunately, family members often keep their anger inside, never allowing their loved one to share in that anger. Or, they may direct their anger at others.

Family members may lash out at the medical providers for not catching the illness in time. They may become angry with friends and other family members for not being supportive enough. They may be angry that their financial situation is now a disaster.

Anger is often viewed as a negative emotion, but the fact is, anger is healthy—as long as it is vented and then let go.

Bargaining

Another of Kübler-Ross's stages is *bargaining*. During this stage the patient may make promises in return for the situation going away. "If only I can be cured, I'll spend my life doing good." Such bargaining is an attempt to buy time, to forestall the inevitable. "It will be okay to die if I can just live to see my daughter married." "I'll devote all my time to my family if I can just see my children grow up." "I'll give my life to God if I can live just a few more years."

Family members, too, may make bargains. "If only Dad can live until Timmy graduates, it will be okay." "If only Mom can get better, I'll be the best daughter in the world." Bargaining helps us believe that we can do something to make the situation better. It gives us a sense of control.

Depression

Depression—a numbing, sometimes debilitating sadness—is another stage of dying A dark cloud of gloom covers everything. "It's useless. I have nothing to live for." Your loved one will feel like she is in a deep, dark hole, with no hope of digging her way out. During this stage, the patient may become withdrawn. She may move slowly, have no appetite, and appear to not care about anything. Visitors may not be welcome.

We sometimes use the word *depression* when we really mean sadness. Depression and sadness are not the same. With sadness, there is still room to experience laughter, joy, and hope. This is not the case with depression. Depression is much more intense than sadness, and is often related to chemical changes in the body triggered by the illness or medication. Fortunately, depression can often be treated.

If you think your loved one is depressed, notify the doctor, hospice nurse, social worker, or other health professional. Signs of severe depression include

- Chronic sadness, anxiety, and complaints of feeling "empty."

- Frequent crying.

- Expressions of guilt, helplessness, hopelessness, and worthlessness.

- Increased alcohol consumption or drug use (including prescription drugs).

- Thoughts of suicide or a suicide attempt.

Family members, too, may become depressed. "I can't go on like this. I have no life of my own." If both the patient and family members are depressed at the same time, the hospice team can be of great assistance, identifying the depression so it can be treated, as well as listening and helping the family find and name the hope that is there.

Acceptance

The ultimate goal is to reach the stage of *acceptance*—a readiness for death. Given time and loving assistance, the patient may come to accept death. Anger and sadness fade. It is not a happy stage, but one of calmness. "It's okay." "I am ready." "I've had a good life, and I love you all. You'll all be fine when I'm gone." The person is at peace.

Family members may also come to acceptance, especially if their loved one has already accepted her own death. "We are so fortunate to have her in our lives." "We'll still have happy times." "This journey will soon be over." Family members who accept the impending death are less likely to seek out and agree to heroic medical interventions. They are more likely to honor their loved one's desire to die with dignity. It is a time to acknowledge the end of a life, knowing that the relationship will live on in memories.

THE REALITY OF DYING

Although some individuals may go through these five stages in the order they are presented, most do not. As Kübler-Ross made clear, this is a model to help understand the dying process. In reality, some patients may experience only one or two of the stages. And they may go back and forth between stages, being angry one day and depressed the next. Acceptance may occur and then disappear.

The way that people live their lives can predict the way they will die. A person who has denied adversity throughout life is likely to also deny death. A person who has faced adversity with anger may face death with anger, too. Likewise, a person who tends to compromise in a conflict may stay in the bargaining stage longer than others. Each person is unique.

There is never enough time for all that we want to say or do. It is never really "okay" for someone to die. Don't expect to accept it right away. What is important is to recognize the emotions that accompany the dying process. Each person dies in his or her own way.

In addition to the five classic stages of dying, you and your loved one can expect other emotions, some pleasant, some unpleasant.

Unpleasant Feelings

Although we all will die, it is natural to fight death, to have very negative feelings about it. It is a loss. It is an unknown. It is beyond our control.

When a loved one is dying, or when we are dying, it is normal to fear death, to feel both grief and guilt.

Fear

After absorbing the shock of a terminal illness, most people face fear. Fear of the unknown may be greater than the fear of death itself.

Dying may be the most frightening experience in your life. People who are dying may fear pain, loss of bodily control, and becoming a burden to those they love. They may fear losing their mental capacities or becoming emotionally unstable. They may fear that their appearance will deteriorate. They may have financial worries. They may feel anxious about how their family will get along without them or how much grief their death will cause. Might family members fight over their possessions? Might family members forget them?

People with a terminal illness may fear when and how they will die. Will there be pain? Will they linger? Will they be conscious? Will their loved ones be with them? Will they know when the time comes?

Dying people may dread what will happen to their body after they die—if they will be displayed, if they will decay or burn. They may fear what will happen after death: Is there nothingness? A heaven? A hell? Reincarnation? Might the spirit travel forever, never finding peace?

Fear can cause great stress, making people tense and short-tempered. It can keep them awake at night. It may come and go. Fear can also lead to indecision. Terminally ill people may question their decision to choose hospice rather than continue seeking a cure.

As a caregiver, you may share your loved one's fears. You may also fear the responsibilities you have taken on, wondering whether or not you can fulfill them. You may fear losing emotional control and revealing your own fears to your loved one. You may fear that others think you aren't doing enough. You may worry that you are neglecting your family or other responsibilities in life. You may fear what life will be like without your loved one. You may become painfully aware of your own mortality. You may worry that the decision to accept comfort care, rather than continuing to seek a possible cure, was a mistake. You may dread being present when your loved one dies. "What if I become hysterical?" "What if I panic?" "What if I can't comfort her?" At the same time, you may fear not being there when death comes.

You cannot know the future, but you can prepare for it. You can learn as much about death and dying as possible. You can try to understand. You can face your fears. List them on paper. Talk about them with your loved one and discuss possible solutions.

Enlist the aid of the hospice team, your family, and your friends. Hospice spiritual care providers are trained to help people with these feelings, as are hospice social workers. It is likely that your friends and family share your fears and doubts, and they may be relieved to finally have a chance to discuss them. There's an old saying that if you worry about what might be and wonder what might have been, you will ignore what is. Live life for today, not for yesterday or tomorrow.

When you begin to feel afraid, take deep breaths, relax. Remind yourself that you're doing the best you can, then let the fear go.

Guilt

Guilt is the way we punish ourselves for not being perfect. To your dying loved one, guilt will likely be an additional source of stress. "Why didn't I take better care of myself?" "Why didn't I seek medical help earlier?" "Why did I ignore the symptoms?" "Why didn't I take out more insurance?" "Why didn't we take that vacation?" "Why am I putting my loved ones through this?"

Guilt can also plague caregivers. "Why didn't I insist that she get a physical?" "Why didn't we do more things together when we could?" "Why do I resent all the things I've had to give up to provide this care?" "Why did I yell at her?" "Why am I angry that she is dying, leaving me alone?"

Guilt can be a vicious circle. Don't dwell on the past, on what you should have done. Forgive yourself and think about what you want to do in the future. And don't expect perfection—you will feel guilty if you don't live up to your own expectations. Do your best. Talk about your feelings with your loved one. Ask each other, "What do you want?" Honesty goes a long way toward preventing guilt. Plan together how you and your loved one can resolve the guilt feelings.

Embarrassment and Humiliation

Our society prizes independence and self-reliance. Your loved one was once independent and self-reliant, and if that is lost, she may feel shame. Losing one's independence may feel like a sign of weakness or failure. Your loved one may feel guilty about asking for help and being a burden on you. "I feel so helpless." "I used to be able to take care of my family; now they take care of me." "If I can't be self-sufficient, there's no point in living." "I'm embarrassed to have my spouse clean up after my messes." It can be difficult for your loved one to ask for help. As a caregiver, you must learn to recognize when help is needed, and then gently provide assistance. Your matter-of-fact approach can make things much easier.

Self-Pity

It is completely natural for your loved one to feel self-pity at times. You, the caregiver, may feel it as well. "I just can't handle any more." Furthermore, you both may have regrets. Everyone does. You both have a right to these feelings. It's okay. But self-pity and regret are a waste of your precious time. Forget what you can't change and make right what you can. Forgive each other. Don't let yourself get overwhelmed and worn out. Turn to the hospice team for help.

Grief

Although grief is usually associated with death itself, it occurs throughout the dying process. There are many losses between the moment a terminal diagnosis turns your world upside down and actual death. Grief is, by definition, the reaction to a loss. Grief felt before the death is called anticipatory grief. It causes both physical and psychological pain. The pain and the tears are real. Give grief the attention that is due it.

Your loved one may grieve for her loss of independence, loss of bodily control, or lost dreams. You, as a caregiver, may grieve for these things and more.

However, grief and sadness are only part of the picture. With the help of hospice, you and your loved one can not only reduce these disagreeable emotions, but experience positive feelings as well.

Dealing with Unpleasant Feelings

Many healthcare providers speak extensively about the healing power of laughter, relaxation, and meditation. Although these may not result in a medical miracle, they often result in miracles of attitude adjustment, of people learning to cope with their illness.

Some Things to Try
Following are suggestions for patients and families dealing with unpleasant feelings:

- Listen to one another.

- Acknowledge the value of what the other person says.

- Let your feelings out.

- Plan enjoyable activities together.

- Use deep breathing, relaxation exercises, and meditation. (Your hospice team can teach you these.)

- Reach out for support.

- Ask your loved one to tell a story from her life that was hopeful or wonderful.

- Make a list of things you are grateful for every day.

- Celebrate small victories.

- Smile and laugh.

- Touch and hug.

- Cry.

- Shout or yell as a release when you are alone.

- Be comfortable with silence.

- Concentrate on *being* rather than on *doing*.

- When the question is "Why?" the answer is "I don't know."

- Keep confidentiality.

- Express your love openly.

- Be yourself.

- Rely on your hospice team members.

Call hospice if your loved one is perspiring and extremely restless, complains of increased pain, is unable to breathe, or expresses thoughts of suicide.

Some Things to Avoid
When dealing with unpleasant feelings, remember the following:

- Do not hold feelings in.

- Do not tell your loved one to "cheer up" if she is depressed.

- Do not blame yourself for the situation.

- Do not try to reason your loved one out of seemingly irrational feelings or statements. Show compassion and understanding.

- Do not judge. Accept and support whatever she feels.

- Do not give assistance without first asking if it is wanted.

- Do not offer advice unless asked.

- Do not be afraid to use the words *death* and *dying*.

- Do not use clichés such as "Things could be worse" or "It's all for the best."

Positive Feelings

Hospice celebrates living. It emphasizes the positives in life. Despite all of the unpleasant emotions, you and your loved one, with the support of hospice, can still experience joy, love, hope, and healing.

Humor and Joy in Hospice

You may feel that humor has no place while coping with something as serious as a terminal disease, but in most instances, this is definitely not the case. If your loved one has a sense of humor, help her to keep it. Appreciate it. The story goes that a friend visited W. C. Fields as he lay on his deathbed reading the Bible. When the friend asked why he was reading it, Fields answered, "I'm looking for the loopholes."

Laughing can open your heart. It can take away some of the hurt. Together, you might recall humorous stories from your past.

Kenneth B. Wentzel, author of *To Those Who Need It Most, Hospice Means Hope,* tells the story of a son who asked a minister to come to his home and baptize his mother, who had suffered a stroke. Partially paralyzed, the mother could only manage to grunt yes or no—the effort to speak was just too great for her. But she had written on a pad of paper that she wished to be baptized. Glad to be of service, the minister went to the home. He asked the mother, "Do you renounce your sin and the evil that is in the world?" She grunted and nodded assent. "Do you wish to be baptized into the Christian faith?" Again she grunted and nodded assent. The minister then took the filled glass standing next to a bowl on the end table and poured the contents into the bowl. He proceeded to baptize the mother, offer a prayer, and conclude with a benediction. After he left, the son came into his mother's room and asked if she had been baptized. She grunted, "Yes." When he asked if she was pleased, his mother squared her shoulders and said, "Yes. But the fool used my 7-Up!" and began to laugh. It was a story she probably enjoyed telling to get others to laugh with her.

When your loved one is dying, joy can be an unexpected emotion for both of you. You must allow yourselves to feel it, and you mustn't feel guilty because of it.

Joy is the essence of our being
The light that shines through us
The stars of our own recognition.
It's the sun in our heart that reminds us
Life is as divine on earth as it is in heaven.
It's a candle that lights the darkness.
It's given us to remind us
Who we were before we were born.
The gift is always present.
It only waits for us to know its presence.

—Anonymous

Love and Compassion

Love and compassion are an integral part of hospice. Those who are dying need words and gestures of affection and love. They need to know that they're loved. Affection is life sustaining. The reality of impending death can make us appreciate more fully those we love. Take time to show this love.

Love is unconditional. It is given even though you and your loved one will soon part. And you both need to love yourselves—unconditionally. We can feel love and compassion for someone else only when we feel it for ourselves as well.

Hope

Embrace your hopes throughout the dying process. You can hope for happy times together. You can hope to keep your loved one's pain under control. You can hope that you will love and be loved. You can hope that until death comes, you and your loved one will live your lives fully. If you hope for the things you can control, you can make them come to pass.

Keep hope alive. Hope can give you time to come to terms with the inevitable. It can help protect you when today seems too difficult to face.

RELATIONSHIPS

Many people view terminal illness as a wake-up call to start living life while there is still life to live. Awareness of approaching death offers everyone a rare opportunity to express their true feelings. It's a time for saying, "Thank you," "I love you," "I'm sorry—forgive me," "I forgive you," and "Goodbye" (from the book by Ira Byock, *Four Things That Matter*). Relationships often grow stronger as the patient and family grapple with living while dying. Once a person begins the transition from life to death, the importance of love, forgiveness, and making peace become evident. This is no time for resentment or grudges.

If misunderstandings occur, someone must take the first step to clear them up. It doesn't matter who. No one should let pride or hurt feelings stop them from clarifying a misunderstanding.

Dealing with Conflict

Sometimes, misunderstandings result in conflict, and conflict can be handled in different ways. You and your loved one can ignore the issue, smooth it over, argue about it, or attempt to resolve the issue through discussion and compromise.

Some conflicts are just not worth arguing about. Other times, it is better to get the issue out in the open. You and your loved one must decide: Is the cost of facing the issue worth the reward? For example, a dying mother may want to discuss funeral arrangements, but her daughter, who has not yet come to accept the imminent death, refuses to do so, saying it is premature. The mother must balance the energy she would need to deal with her daughter's resistance with the closure and comfort she would find in making final arrangements. The daughter must balance having to face her own fear about her mother's dying with her desire to please her mother. To have a healthy discussion of the issues involved, both parties must agree that the discussion is "worth it."

People in conflict may behave defensively. For example, patients recently informed their cancer is terminal may refuse to discuss hospice at all, insisting that they aren't really going to die. To deal with this sort of defensive behavior, expect it, acknowledge it, and *try not to intensify it.* Simply listen and nod. Ask your loved one what she knows about the disease. Ask what she knows about hospice. Give your loved one time to come to terms with the circumstances. If you confront your loved one, you may find yourself in a fight or flight situation where neither person is likely to win.

Without effective communication, the most important people in your life may become your greatest source of frustration. When conflicts arise, your hospice team can help. Take advantage of their objective views and their willingness to act as mediators.

SPIRITUAL ISSUES

> *Faith that dying is part of the breathing in and out of the universe, and not an end, facilitates the dying process. Dying is more easily accepted by a person who feels a sunset is not the end of the sun and shedding a body is not the end of life. She or he will likely pass more quickly through the stages of dying—not skipping fear or anger but spending less time with them.*
>
> —Deborah Duda, *Coming Home*

After a terminal diagnosis, many people confront profound spiritual questions about the meaning of their life and death. With hospice, care for the spirit is just as important as care for the body. In fact, the founder of the modern hospice movement, Dr. Cicely Saunders, related sickness and dying to the suffering of Jesus. Her view of spiritual support was deeply rooted in Judeo-Christian belief.

Today's hospice, however, recognizes that different people hold different beliefs. Some are atheists, discounting any higher being. Others embrace a formal, organized religion. Still others have their own personal system of beliefs.

Spiritual support can take many forms, such as a caring relationship with loved ones, an acceptance of mortality, or faith in a higher power. Spiritual support could center on a Supreme Being and an organized religion, or it might avoid the subject of religion altogether. Either way, spiritual support means conveying faith, hope, and love. It means listening to your loved one, acknowledging her uncertainties, and helping her to let go of guilt, regret, and other signs of spiritual pain. If this is difficult to grasp, remember that your hospice team includes a spiritual counselor who can help.

Faith is a key part of spiritual support. Faith lets us feel that all is right, even though we do not understand what is happening or why. Faith reduces our fears and lets us live today more completely. Everyone has faith in something, even if it's simply that the sun will rise in the morning. Faith is what keeps us going despite misfortune.

In taking care of spiritual needs, you and your loved one must strive to achieve peace of mind. Dr. Daniel Tobin's book *Peaceful Dying* describes a simple mind-quieting technique that can help. Imagine putting all your problems—those that still trouble you—onto a raft docked on a river. Pile your problems in. When all your concerns are aboard, gently, lovingly push the raft away so it can float down the river. Watch it drift until it is out of sight. Then, turn away and go about the business of living.

Unresolved conflicts make peace of mind difficult to achieve. You must do what you can to let go of these past conflicts. For example, stop fretting about the past and worrying about the future. Work at living in the present. Forget the notion that you can control everything. Fix what you can, and let the rest go.

Understanding the feelings that accompany death is a step toward accepting them. It will take time. There will be laughter and tears and all the emotions in between. It's natural and normal. Take each day as it comes. Request support from your spiritual care provider if this would be helpful.

3

Being a Caregiver:
One Day at a Time

*Taking care of terminally ill patients is a privilege
and a gift which teaches us not only about dying,
but about living.*

—Elisabeth Kübler-Ross

*"What a glorious day," Ella exclaimed. Before hospice she had never
really thought about each day as something precious, but all that had
changed. She was pleased that the sun was shining so she and John
could sit outside together for a while. As she counted out the medications for the day, she thought ahead to when their son, Tim, would be
over to watch a video with John while she took a few hours for herself—something she hadn't done for quite a while. Today she would
get her hair done and read her favorite magazine. Checking over her
"to-do" list, Ella felt satisfaction knowing she was doing her best, with
the support of family, friends, and hospice.*

Caregiving may be the hardest thing you will ever do. For instance,
caring for your dying loved one may compete with other responsibilities: children, work, or both. Even so, most people who have
done it say the challenge is worthwhile.

Being a caregiver allows you to show your loved one how much he
means to you. It is a chance to give something back. It is a chance to
express your true feelings through your actions and your presence.

As a caregiver you will assume many roles: family spokesperson, patient advocate, information center, and hospice team captain. You will look out for your loved one's best interests, seeing that his physical, emotional, and spiritual needs are met.

You will have much to learn and many new responsibilities to fulfill. You will watch your loved one's physical condition deteriorate despite your best efforts. But of all the challenges you will face on this journey, dealing with change may be the most difficult.

FACING CHANGE

> *All changes involve loss, just as all losses require change.*
>
> —Robert Neimeyer

In the coming days, weeks, and months, you will experience many changes. Perhaps you've already seen a change in family dynamics. You will delegate responsibilities to family members, and you will open your home to strangers—members of the hospice team.

Changes like these evoke the conflicting emotions of fear and hope, anxiety and relief. Change threatens our self-esteem and forces us to face new challenges. It is natural to resist change. After all, change pushes us into the unknown, when we are far more comfortable with the status quo.

You, your loved one, and the rest of your family will need to work toward accepting change. One of the biggest changes will probably occur in your relationship with other family members.

Changes in Family Relationships

It's important for you to ask for the help you need. Although you may be the primary caregiver, other family members should also be involved in caregiving. If you're the main caregiver, you may feel taken for granted, and your resentment may build. This may lead to conflicts between the needs of your loved one and the needs of the rest of the family. These conflicts may be difficult to resolve. The hospice team is there to answer any questions that you have and may help facilitate family conferences. Some family members will be less involved in caregiving than others. They may live in another city, have young children at home, or be unable to leave a job. Expect conflicts to arise when one person takes on most of the work while others watch from the sidelines.

When adult children are involved, they sometimes regress to their earlier sibling relationships, keeping tally on who's doing more chores and who's receiving more privileges. Consider the following suggestions for handling family relationships with minimum stress and maximum efficiency:

- State clearly what you can and cannot do.

- Be forthright and honest. Don't manipulate one family member by dropping hints to another.

- Be dependable. If you say you're going to do something, do it.

- Be forgiving and ask for forgiveness if you need it.

- Turn to friends if your family cannot offer the support you need.

Let your loved one participate in his own care as much as possible. This will help your loved one maintain a sense of control and independence.

Family conferences are an excellent means of resolving conflict, allowing open discussion on how responsibilities might be shared. This is especially important for supporting the primary caregiver. Specific tasks can be assigned according to individual schedules and abilities. These assignments may be modified as family members' circumstances change. The hospice social worker can arrange for appropriate hospice team members to attend your family conferences. If you need to, alternate visiting periods for family members who cannot resolve their conflicts.

Opening Your Home to Others

Home is more than a shelter from the elements. Home is where people go to escape the worries and frustrations of life. However, when someone is dying there, home becomes the center of worry and frustration.

At this intensely personal time, you may find it difficult to have the hospice staff, who are strangers at first, in your home. It may help to know that many hospice workers joined hospice after caring for a loved one of their own. They are committed to helping others who are facing death. By participating in such an intense, intimate time in a family's life, hospice workers often become valued allies.

ATTENDING TO PHYSICAL NEEDS

When you first think about caregiving, you may focus on tending to physical needs: preparing meals, helping your loved one in and out of a bed or chair, managing symptoms like nausea and pain, giving medications, assisting with bathing and dressing, and managing the household.

Indeed, these are awesome responsibilities. Caregiver training comes strictly on the job and under duress. Hospice support is extremely important because most people have little experience in caring for a dying loved one.

Keeping your loved one physically comfortable is an important part of hospice care. The nursing staff can teach you common caregiving techniques based on your abilities, the patient's needs, and the physical setup of the home.

As a caregiver you will learn to manage hygiene, nutrition, sleep problems, and pain control. You will learn to identify emerging problems and to propose solutions. You may also help your loved one make financial decisions and funeral preparations. Each day will bring new learning experiences and new challenges.

MAKING DECISIONS

Caregivers are involved in day-to-day problem solving and decision making. Some of these decisions can be quite difficult. For example, what if your loved one becomes mentally impaired due to the illness or medication? What if he wants to stop taking the pain medication, saying, "I want to know what's going on around me, even if stopping my pills brings back the pain." What do you do? Do you agree? Do you try to sneak the pills into food or drink? How do you decide? Does your loved one really mean that he wants the pain? Ethical questions like these should be discussed as early as possible. However, if the situation arises, and you have not talked about it beforehand, try to think how your loved one would have felt before the illness. And remember, the hospice team can help with decisions like this.

THE EMOTIONAL ROLLER COASTER

Caring for the dying is an emotionally charged activity. It is a time when new levels of love, understanding, and appreciation may be reached between you and your loved one.

The dying process brings intense emotions that require exceptional coping skills. Studies have shown that people are far less stressed by the practical, financial, and physical aspects of caregiving than they are by the emotional aspects.

Powerful thoughts and emotions will overlap and change daily—even hourly—with the circumstances. Anticipating these feelings will help reduce the fear and loss that is so common when a loved one is dying.

Anger is an especially difficult emotion for caregivers. You may find yourself angry at your loved one for placing this responsibility on you or for leaving you before it's time. Anger is a normal, healthy reaction to any perceived threat.

For hospice patients, anger is usually a response to feelings of fear, helplessness, and frustration. The anger of a dying person is one of the most difficult emotions for caregivers to confront. In fact, caregivers are often the target of hostility. Patients can get very demanding. They've lost so much control in their lives that they sometimes try to control the people around them.

For most patients, lashing out actually means, "Why did this have to happen to me?" It represents rage at having to die and sometimes anger that family members will survive. In some cases, patients do not realize they are acting differently. Medication, or the disease itself, may aggravate their anger.

Many caregivers won't respond to a patient's anger as they normally would. They know their loved one is extremely vulnerable and dependent, so they stifle their feelings until the hurt becomes unbearable. Then they explode, often saying things they don't mean or behaving in ways that unfairly punish those who are closest to them.

Anger is to be expected when a loved one is dying. Families may wish to discuss anger and other emotions with a clergy member, the hospice spiritual care provider, or the hospice social worker. Share your fears and frustrations with members of the hospice team. They won't take your anger personally, and they won't think any less of you. They are there to help your entire family cope.

Even when death is certain, there is room for hope. In hospice, hope is redefined. You might hope for a life without pain or discomfort, or for a meaningful, loving time with family and friends. Some people find it helpful to adopt a "just-in-case" approach: They maintain their hope for a cure or miraculous recovery, but, just in case it doesn't happen, they are prepared for death. This allows them to hold on to their hopes while accepting reality.

SPIRITUAL SUPPORT

Spiritual questions about why are we here and what happens after death are not easily answered. If your loved one's faith offers answers and comfort, support that faith. If, on the other hand, your loved one is troubled by fear of the unknown, you can help by sharing your own questions and uncertainties, validating that his concerns are normal and reasonable. The hospice team can help with spiritual questions, too, bringing comfort in this difficult time.

COMMUNICATION

As a caregiver, it is important that you communicate openly and honestly with your loved one. Don't assume a false cheerfulness. Your loved one will see through it every time. Reassure him that you are willing to listen and to talk about all aspects of the illness— even though it may be hard for both of you.

Create a climate that encourages the sharing of emotions. Help your loved one talk about anxiety and depression. Explain your own needs, and discuss how your loved one can make caregiving easier. For example, if your loved one experiences pain, you need to know as soon as that pain begins. If your loved one waits until the pain is severe, it will be much harder to manage.

Don't feel you have to be perpetually entertaining or fill every moment with meaning. You'll exhaust yourself and your loved one. Let your loved one share thoughts and feelings on his own terms. Remember, sharing does not always mean talking. Some people are more comfortable writing about feelings or expressing them without words. Hospice patients want to share many things, but they may not share them all with you. Encourage your loved one to talk privately with whomever he wishes.

Understand when your loved one doesn't follow your advice or resists your offers to handle personal matters. It is natural to want to retain independence and control. Allow your loved one every opportunity to make decisions, no matter how small, from choices about meals to which clothes to wear. Phrase your questions in a way that encourages an honest answer, such as "What can I prepare for you that will taste good right now?" Finally, include your loved one in choices about medical treatment. Decisions like these will affect your loved one's quality of life, and he must be allowed to participate in these decisions.

MAINTAINING QUALITY OF LIFE

Make every effort to maintain your loved one's dignity and independence. Set a routine that becomes comfortable for both of you.

Then, add at least one break in the routine each day. Share meals, television programs, reading, music, photo albums, and quiet moments outdoors. You might even work on a special project together.

ATTENDING TO CHILDREN'S NEEDS

Children dealing with terminal illness and death have special needs. Talk to them on their level. Answer their questions honestly. Have them spend time with your loved one. If the children are old enough, let them help in caregiving. Assign them simple tasks such as watching a favorite television program with their loved one. Ask for their help with emptying the trash and other household tasks.

These children's lives have been disrupted. They may resent the time you spend with your dying loved one. Here are some suggestions for helping children cope when a loved one is dying:

- Take time to talk to each child individually.

- Ask children what they already know about the illness.

- Be honest, upbeat, and realistic.

- Help children focus on activities they can still do with their loved one.

- Explain that the illness is not their fault and that illnesses are never caused by a person or an event.

- Teach children how to hope for things other than a cure.

- Assure children that the illness is not "catching."

- It's okay to say, "I don't know."

- It's okay to cry.

- Let children know there will always be someone to take care of them.

- Be prepared for anger.

- Encourage children to talk openly about their feelings.

- Do not whisper.

- Ask children if they understand what you have said.

- Keep children updated.

- Make only promises you can keep.

- Reassure children of your unconditional love.

- Encourage children to write or draw pictures of how they feel.

- If you have children living at home, it is extremely important to make home a happy place.

Children's grief may take months and years to resolve. Ask your hospice team to suggest age-appropriate resources to help you and your children discuss death.

MAINTAINING BALANCE

No one can sincerely try to help another without helping himself.

—Charles Dudley Warner

The often-repeated advice to caregivers is to take care of *themselves.* Eat right. Exercise. Get plenty of sleep each night. Take time out to go to a movie or get out of the house. But how?

Caring for a dying person can be physically and emotionally

draining. Even with considerable help from hospice, family, and friends, you are ultimately responsible for helping your loved one complete his earthly journey.

Your well-being is crucial. Caring for yourself is not a sign of selfishness. It is a matter of replenishing yourself and staying healthy so you can give your loved one the best care possible. Like a long-distance runner, you must preserve your strength and pace yourself. You may be overextending yourself if you feel

- Restless.

- Depressed.

- Trapped.

- Obsessed with your caregiving responsibilities.

- Deeply resentful of your loved one or other family members.

- Indispensable, as if the whole world rests on your shoulders.

To make it through these difficult days, recognize your limitations. Preserve and foster your strength. You might try behaviors that came naturally to you as a child:

- Say "no" when you feel like it.

- Do what you want to do.

- Ask for what you need.

- Refuse to second-guess what others want.

- Refuse to do work that someone else should be doing.

- Seek out people you like to be with.

- Stay away from difficult people if you can.

A problem that many caregivers face is sleep deprivation. This often is due to the erratic sleep patterns of your loved one. Try to get at least six hours of sleep each night, and take naps while your loved one is sleeping during the day.

Make a point of getting out of the house periodically. Other family members or friends can take over while you're away—sometimes they are just waiting to be asked. Give yourself—as a caregiver—permission to ask for help. In addition, hospice has trained volunteers who can give you a break. Remember, you are only one person, and you cannot do everything. Some form of respite is essential in prolonged caregiving. If you are becoming exhausted, let the hospice team know. They may suggest changes in the care plan to meet everyone's needs.

CAREGIVING AS A PARTNERSHIP

Caregiving is not an "all or nothing" activity. You need not take full responsibility—nor should you leave the entire responsibility to others. It is a partnership that includes your loved one, your family, and the hospice team.

Caregiving can be overwhelming, especially if you try to do it all yourself. That's why a team approach is essential. Although one person may be the main caregiver, a variety of responsibilities can be rotated among family members, friends, hospice professionals, and volunteers.

All members of the immediate family, as well as close friends, can help with caregiving. Specific roles may vary, but the fact that friends and family are doing *something* lets them feel they are contributing.

Some friends will offer to help. Gratefully acknowledge this offer, accept it, and then suggest some options. They might schedule regular time with your loved one, giving you some time to yourself. They might clean the house, do yard work, or drive the children to school, lessons, and other activities. They can shop, run errands, lend an ear, or give you a hug. Keep a written list of tasks and activities that people could help with so you don't have to rely on your memory when someone calls to offer assistance.

Hospice professionals and volunteers can help family members and friends identify caregiving roles. The role each person plays must be appropriate for that individual. The goal is to do all you can—not more than you can—to care for your loved one.

Many caregivers are reluctant to share caregiving responsibilities. They convince themselves that only they can care for their loved one, that no one else can do it as well. The fact is, the challenges of caregiving are simply too great. You can't do it all—not indefinitely, at any rate.

The following guidelines will help you care for yourself while caring for your loved one:

- Talk to your loved one about his needs and expectations.

- Discuss backup plans in case you are unable to fulfill these needs and expectations. Include family members if possible.

- Confide in other family members who will offer suggestions and support.

- Ask the hospice social worker to help you access community resources. Homemakers, pastoral ministers, respite volunteers, meals-on-wheels, and the like may be available through local churches and synagogues, community centers, and county agencies.

- When your loved one is resting, use this opportunity to do something for yourself. Exercise, phone a supportive friend, pray, meditate, read, attend a support group, or just rest.

- Take advantage of offers for help from family, friends, neighbors, and professionals.

- If you can afford it, hire someone to spend a day watching your loved one so you can take a break or focus on other responsibilities. If your loved one is up a lot at night, hire someone to stay awake with him so you can get a full night's sleep.

- Understand that you and your loved one will experience a roller coaster of emotions. This is normal.

- Try not to feel guilty or personally responsible if your loved one is unusually critical or angry. As an illness progresses, patients often feel most comfortable expressing their frustrations to the people closest to them.

- Make full use of your hospice team.

- It is normal to feel sad, afraid, and alone at times. Just remember to ask for help and to take one day at a time.

How the Hospice Team Can Help

Registered nurses, home health aides, social workers, therapists, spiritual care providers, music and massage therapists, and other professionals are available to lighten the caregiving load. They can provide physical or emotional relief, answer questions, and offer support. They will help ensure your loved one receives the best possible care.

Each week, volunteers can give caregivers a short break from their responsibilities. The hospice team may schedule an aide to periodically attend to your loved one's personal needs throughout the week. Or, depending on the patient's Medicare or insurance benefits, respite care occasionally may be offered in a healthcare facility.

Members of the hospice team will let caregivers know what changes to expect and what events will likely occur as the person dies. Hospice also offers spiritual support to help make sense of the dying process and to give caregivers the strength to carry on.

Daily Caregiving:
Each Day a Gift

*Ella vividly remembered the day she and John decided on hospice—
on comfort care at home. She recalled how the hospice team helped
her and the family prepare the home for caregiving and how overwhelming it all seemed at first. But now that they could focus on living, each day was treasured. The routine of caring for physical,
spiritual, and emotional needs was comfortable and comforting.
John, the family, the hospice professionals and volunteers, and Ella
were truly becoming a team.*

SETTING UP THE HOME

> *Happiness consists more in small conveniences or
> pleasures that occur every day, than in great pieces
> of good fortune that happen but seldom.*
>
> —Benjamin Franklin

Whether or not your loved one is being discharged from the hospital, the decision to provide hospice care requires a transition
plan. As you make your transition plan, your key considerations
should be *patient comfort* and *ease of caregiving*.

   As you prepare your home for hospice care, you will want to
consider your loved one's ability to get around. Focus on safety,

convenience, accessibility, and cleanliness, and try to maintain a cheerful and private environment. *As a general rule, stay with the familiar whenever possible.*

With these considerations in mind, ask yourself the following questions: Where will your loved one's room be? Do stairs pose a problem? Can you install handrails on stairways? Can you position a walker at the top and bottom of the stairs? Is the bathroom accessible? The television? The phone? Are there loose rugs that might be tripped over? If your loved one will be in a wheelchair, is there space to maneuver? After looking at the big picture, carefully examine each room your loved one might use.

The Bedroom

Ideally, your loved one will keep her own bedroom. However, if stairs prevent this, you will have to make a decision: Can your loved one stay in a first-floor guest room, a portion of the family room, or a screened-off section of the living room? No matter what you decide, try to keep the home as normal as possible for the entire family.

The next decision is what kind of bed your loved one will use—a hospital bed or a normal bed. With a hospital bed, you can raise the head or foot of the bed. You can lower the entire bed to help your loved one get in and out, or you can raise the bed for feeding, bathing, and other activities. These beds also have side rails that can be raised and lowered. Most hospice programs can provide a hospital bed, or you can rent one. A disadvantage to having a hospital bed is that it's not the patient's own bed. Hospital beds also make cuddling more difficult since they are twin size.

A normal bed will work for most people receiving hospice care. The bed should have easy access from either side. A firm mattress will be needed to prevent your loved one from slipping off the edge and falling. (If necessary, you can place a bed board underneath the mattress to make it firm.) You may be able to install side rails. You might also attach bars or a trapeze (secure, hanging bars for grabbing) to the bed to help your loved one get in and out. A footstool with rubber feet and a nonskid surface might help, too. Devices are available to keep covers off the feet—these are placed at the foot of the bed. If your loved one can no longer leave the bed, you might want to place a second mattress on top of the first to enhance comfort and assist caregiving activities. The ideal height is usually between 30 and 32 inches from the floor.

Have an ample supply of sheets and blankets in case the bed needs to be changed several times in one day. Hospital beds are twin size, but any size sheet will work. Also a foam mattress may make the bed more comfortable if your loved one will be spending lots of time in it. A washable mattress pad is also a good idea. Provide three or four good pillows to keep your loved one comfortable. Triangular pillows can be placed under the knees for better circulation. An over-the-bed tray or raised lap tray can be used if your loved one will be eating meals or working on projects in bed. If your loved one cannot walk to the bathroom, you might provide a bedside commode. If this is too difficult, a bedpan, urinal or catheter could be used.

A sturdy nightstand or bedside caddy can hold glasses, tissues, books, remote controls, and the like. Try to keep your loved one's personal treasures in plain view. This can be reassuring and comforting. If hospital-style gowns are easier for both of you, consider slitting the back of favorite nightgowns or nightshirts and sewing ties on. The same can be done with favorite dresses and shirts.

Make your loved one's room as cheerful, bright, comfortable, accessible, safe, and convenient as possible. It should be well ventilated and kept at a comfortable, constant temperature. Windows are preferred—you might consider placing a bird feeder outside the window or perhaps a soothing wind chime. Pull dark shades over the windows when your loved one wants to sleep. A recliner, glider, or comfortable chair is another nice feature. Be sure it is easy to get in and out of. You might also bring in a chair or two for visitors.

If possible, provide a telephone, a TV, and a remote control. Make sure your loved one can alert you if needed (using a bell, whistle, intercom, or "baby monitor," for example). If space permits, you might set up an aquarium. Plants and flowers will add to the room's ambiance. Keep the room tidy, but not annoyingly so. If any changes are to be made, discuss them first with your loved one.

The Bathroom

Bathrooms can be dangerous, especially for someone who is weak and unsteady. If your loved one can attend to grooming and toileting, make the bathroom as safe, accessible, and convenient as possible. The door should be wide enough to accommodate a wheelchair or walker, if these will be used. It should open and close easily. You might consider removing the locks.

Easing on or off the toilet can sometimes be difficult. If this is the case, a portable commode can be adjusted and placed over the toilet. Hospice staff can assist with ordering this.

To make bathing easier, use a bath chair in the bathtub or shower. If your loved one has trouble getting in and out of the bathtub, you might obtain a transfer bench. Your loved one can sit on the bench outside the tub and swing her legs over to the inside. If your loved one will be using the shower, consider replacing glass doors with a shower curtain. A hand-held shower hose with a long, flexible tube makes showering easier. If a bath mat is used, make sure it has nonslip backing.

Both the bathtub and shower should have grab bars and safety rails. The floor of the tub or shower should have a bath mat or safety strips. A tub or shower caddy can hold washcloths, soap, shampoo, and other items.

If your loved one needs to sit while shaving, combing hair, or brushing teeth, be sure the mirror is at a convenient height. Also, make a signaling device available in case she needs help.

Our society views activities performed in the bathroom as very private and personal. Your loved one may be embarrassed if she needs assistance bathing or toileting. Assure your loved one that the body is *not* the person. If you are very matter-of-fact about it, your loved one will find it easier to accept your help.

The Kitchen

Because the kitchen is often the center of family activity, it should be accessible to your loved one if possible. If the family eats there, make certain a wheelchair can fit at the table. Use nonskid wax on the floor, and secure any scatter rugs.

Be sensitive to the odors created when preparing and cooking food. They may not smell pleasant to your loved one, so check with her to understand what she can tolerate.

The Living Room and Family Room

If your loved one is mobile, provide a safe, convenient, and easily accessible chair in the living room or family room. An adjustable recliner may be particularly comfortable. Keep a small pillow, a footstool, and a blanket with the chair, and consider attaching a swing-away, self-storing tray for your loved one's belongings.

EQUIPMENT AND SUPPLIES

Your hospice nurse and social worker can help you determine which equipment and supplies you will need for your loved one. Many items are provided by hospice. Some are covered by insurance or the Medicare hospice benefit; others are available through organizations such as the American Cancer Society. Be sure to ask the hospice team before purchasing any equipment or supplies.

Equipment

bath bench or chair
bedpan
commode
crutches
hospital bed
oxygen equipment/tanks
radio
safety rails for tub and toilet
side rails for bed
signaling device
television
trapeze for bed
tray (stand-up or over-the-bed)
urinal
walker
wheelchair

Supplies

adult diapers
dishes with suction-cup bottoms
sipper cups
dressings
eyedropper
gloves, disposable
heating pad
large-faced calendar/clock
lip balm
lotions and creams for the body
medication containers
medications
nonslip socks, slippers
pajamas—extra
pillows—extra
sheets—extra
thermometer
waterproof pads for bed and chair

Getting your home ready for hospice care is a challenge. Your next challenge is to list all the tasks that must be done and who might be able to do them. Remember that hospice is a team effort.

SETTING UP THE TEAM

A good way to get organized is to divide a three-ring binder into four sections: hospice team, care needs, household tasks, and expenses. This notebook should be readily accessible to all team members. You might also use your computer or PDA to help organize this information.

Team Members

You should display the twenty-four-hour hospice number near the main telephone. In your notebook, list all members of the hospice team and their phone numbers. Then list family members and friends who have volunteered to help. Include all other phone numbers you might need, such as the doctor, pharmacy, or medical supply company. Keep a calendar so team member visits can be documented and coordinated.

Physical Care Needs

First, list all the physical assistance you think your loved one may need (getting in and out of bed, dressing, toileting, bathing and grooming, eating, taking medications, exercising, and the like). Next, hold a caregiver meeting to set a daily schedule. Determine who will provide assistance and when. You and your loved one might also decide when visitors are most welcome. The schedule should be flexible, as circumstances are likely to change.

In your caregiver notebook, reserve space for jotting down notes about care provided, symptoms noted, food and fluid intake, and other comments. For each medication, record the name, dose, date started, date discontinued, purpose, and instructions.

Emotional and Spiritual Needs

Physical needs are easy to list, but emotional and spiritual needs can be more difficult. Remember, comfort is a spiritual value. Ask your loved one, "What would bring you comfort today?" Try to arrange activities that will bring comfort and meet your loved one's emotional and spiritual needs. Regardless of religion, we are all spiritual beings.

Don't hesitate to talk over spiritual concerns with the hospice spiritual care provider. You might even ask members of your loved one's faith community to come to the house for support and prayer.

Household Tasks

Hospice volunteers and home health aides may help with some housekeeping tasks, but they won't be able to manage the entire household. This is usually the responsibility of the primary care-giver, family, and friends. Do not be afraid to ask for help. You must take care of yourself so that you can care for your loved one. List the household tasks in your notebook, then hold a family meeting (inviting members of the hospice team) to discuss who might help and how. Consider meal planning, preparation, and cleanup; cleaning and dusting; laundry; shopping; pet care; and errands. If there are young children, their needs should also be considered.

Expenses

Time tends to blur for most caregivers, so good record keeping is important. In addition to medications, you will want to keep a careful record of expenses. Some expenses may be reimbursable through Medicare or your insurance; others may be tax deductible.

For each expense, note the date, item, purpose, cost, and whether it was prescribed by a doctor. Keep your receipts for all caregiving expenses in a separate folder.

COMING HOME

If your loved one is being discharged from a hospital, you will need to consider her mode of transportation. Will your loved one require an ambulance or is a family vehicle appropriate? If possible, make this decision with your loved one.

It is best to pack up your loved one's flowers, cards, gifts, and personal belongings a day or two ahead of time. This way, you can give full attention to your loved one on the day of discharge, and you can have her bedroom ready in advance. In the meantime, you might want to meet with the doctor, hospital social worker, discharge nurse, and members of the hospice team to establish a care plan. They will probably give you instructions for meals, rest, bathing, and medications.

The move may be hard on your loved one. If the trip is long, you might ask the physician about a sedative in case your loved one becomes overly anxious or agitated.

DAILY PHYSICAL CARE

> *The caregiver who cradles your feet, makes soft*
> *rings for your heels, removes wrinkles and crumbs*
> *from the undersheet, sponges you off with a skilled*
> *hand, she is an angel from Heaven.*
>
> **(a doctor as he lay dying)**
> —Deborah Whiting Little

Initially, your loved one may be able to do most things on her own. As her disease progresses and weakness sets in, however, it is likely that more assistance will be needed. Always explain what you are doing and why. Try not to be compulsive. If your loved one doesn't want a shampoo, it can usually wait until tomorrow. A home health aide may be available to help with personal care.

Bathing

Cleanliness helps a person maintain dignity and a sense of control. When bathing your loved one, pay special attention to the genital and underarm areas, where odor-causing bacteria are likely to accumulate. To prevent dry skin, use warm water instead of hot, choose a soap without lots of perfumes and additives, and rinse the soap off thoroughly. Watch for changes in the skin, such as red spots or areas sensitive to the touch. Careful washing or bathing is especially important after incidents where there is a loss of control of bladder or bowels.

After every bath, dry the skin thoroughly, paying special attention to any folds in the skin. Apply a lotion or cream with a water-soluble base, rubbing in gently but thoroughly. Avoid alcohol-based lotions or creams, as these will dry the skin. Consider using baking soda instead of deodorant.

Grooming

Your loved one may need help shaving. Also, her hair should be brushed and combed daily. This not only stimulates the scalp, it improves appearance and morale. Hair should be washed as needed. If your loved one is bedridden, you might consider a "no rinse" shampoo such as those used in hospitals. You simply pour the shampoo on the hair, massage it in, and towel dry. If your loved one prefers a more traditional shampoo, place a pillow in a plastic bag, cover it with a towel, and put it under your loved one's neck. Keep a shallow pan of warm water near her head. Support the head with one hand and begin shampooing with the other. Use the pan to catch the water as you wash your loved one's hair. Consider using a hair dryer afterward so your loved one doesn't get chilled. Some caregivers choose to have a beautician or barber come to the home regularly.

Fingernails and toenails should be cut and kept clean. A manicure or pedicure could be a special treat.

If you have trouble grooming your loved one, ask the hospice home health aide for assistance. An aide can help with shaving, shampooing, and other activities.

Skin Care

The skin is our largest organ. It controls our body temperature and conveys comforting sensations such as hugging. It gets thinner and less elastic as a person ages. Skin may become wrinkled and dry. Skin problems may result from cold, wind, sun, hot water, poor nutrition, lack of exercise, incontinence, or remaining in one position for prolonged periods of time. When going outside on a sunny day, your loved one should wear long sleeves, perhaps a hat, and sunscreen on exposed skin.

Dry Skin. A lack of oil and water in the skin will cause it to become rough and flaky. Dry skin may result from dehydration, heat, cold, radiation therapy, or chemotherapy. Water-soluble skin creams can help. Dry skin may lead to another common problem—itching.

Itching. Itching may be caused by dry skin, toxins in the blood, allergies, medications, depression, or anxiety. The normal reaction to an itch is to scratch it. This usually makes the itch worse, leading to an itch-scratch cycle. In addition to using lotions and creams and avoiding hot water, your loved one shouldn't over bathe and should avoid tight clothing. Ask the hospice nurse about topical medications to relieve the itching.

Pressure ulcers. Pressure ulcers, formerly known as bedsores, may be a persistent problem, causing pain and misery. Pressure ulcers occur when an area of the skin loses its blood supply so nutrients and oxygen can't get to it. Confinement or inactivity results in pressure on certain parts of the body. Most susceptible are areas where the skin is close to the bone: the back of the head, shoulder blades, spine, elbows, tailbone, hipbone, heels, and ankles. They may also appear if the patient is left in urine or feces too long.

To prevent pressure ulcers, your loved one should move or be moved every two to three hours. Exercise or simply turning in bed is very important. If your loved one is bedridden, she might be able to sit up and dangle her legs over the side several times a day to increase blood circulation. If in a wheelchair, your loved one might lift up her body every half hour or so. If your loved one is immobile, your hospice nurse or home health aide can show you how to turn her body by using a draw sheet.

If your loved one has a favorite position, she may resist other positions. Explain the importance of lying in different positions to prevent joint stiffness, promote circulation, and avoid pressure ulcers. The more movement, the better.

To keep skin from touching skin and causing pressure, put a pillow between the legs and a towel between the arms and the body. Make sure the sheets are dry, wrinkle free, and crumb free. Change the sheets whenever they are dirty, wet, or sweaty. This may happen several times in one day or once every two or three days. To help keep the bed clean and dry, sprinkle the sheets with cornstarch and use a rubberized flannel undersheet. A dense foam mattress or an air mattress can relieve pressure on the skin. Do not use a plastic or foam donut to relieve pressure. To prevent heel ulcers, relieve pressure of the heels on the mattress by supporting the lower legs with a pillow, keeping the heels suspended above the mattress.

Massage the susceptible areas of the body, and use a good moisturizing lotion. Watch for redness, especially in areas where bones protrude. If the redness persists, tell your hospice nurse. If pressure sores occur, the nurse can explain how to care for them. Because they are ulcers, they are very slow to heal. Some pressure sores require special solutions and dressing supplies. Regular bathing will help reduce the odor that often accompanies pressure ulcers.

Changes in Skin Color. Internal changes may cause changes in skin color. A yellowing of the skin may indicate liver problems. If the skin takes on a bluish cast, your loved one may be having breathing difficulties. Changes in skin color may indicate that the illness is progressing, or they may be side effects of radiation or chemotherapy. While these changes should be noted, they require no action.

Wounds. Wounds are usually caused by illness, injury, or an incision during surgery. Sometimes they are a side effect of radiation therapy. For some wounds, dressings must be changed frequently. Your hospice nurse will instruct you in wound care and help you get the appropriate supplies.

Stomas. A stoma is a surgically cut opening in the body to replace a natural opening that has become obstructed or has been removed. The three most common stomas are a colostomy in the colon, a urostomy in the bladder, and a tracheostomy in the airway. If your loved one requires a stoma, your hospice nurse can teach you how to care for it.

Dental Care

The condition of our mouth and teeth affect how we feel, eat, look, and talk. We all need to brush and floss our teeth at least once a day, preferably after every snack or meal. If toothpaste is too messy for your loved one, you might try using a toothette, a spongy swab containing special cleansers as directed by your hospice nurse.

Mouth Care

People with terminal illnesses might encounter a dry mouth, tongue fissures, and bleeding gums. These conditions can be painful and can also cause bad breath. Frequent rinsing is recommended. Avoid commercial mouthwashes—the alcohol they contain may irritate mouth tissue. Instead, use diluted solutions of salt or baking soda in warm water. Many people tend to mouth breathe toward the end of life, and using oral swabs every four hours is important. Be careful that your loved one does not bite off the sponge.

You can apply petroleum jelly to the tongue or dry lips, unless your loved one receives oxygen. Petroleum-based products (such as regular Vaseline) should not be used on or around anyone receiving oxygen because it is a highly flammable material. Instead, for dry lips and tongue, apply K-Y jelly or another non-petroleum-based product. Dentures should receive their normal care. It may seem like a bother, but dentures can be very important to your loved one's dignity and self-image.

Foot Care

When a person is inactive, her feet may suffer. Feet need activity for circulation. You might encourage exercises for the feet, moving them in a circular motion. Massage the feet and keep them soft with a lanolin lotion. To soften calluses, wrap your loved one's feet in a warm, wet towel covered in plastic for fifteen to thirty minutes. You might also consider medicated foot powder.

Eye Care

For some terminally ill patients, the ability to blink becomes impaired. If this occurs, artificial tears—as well as a warm washcloth over the eyes—might help. If the ability to blink is completely lost, your hospice nurse might suggest eye patches.

CARING FOR SYMPTOMS

Palliative care, or comfort care, means attending to every ache and pain while empathizing with anything that causes your loved one embarrassment or loss of dignity. The symptoms most distressing to your loved one may involve the loss of control over bodily functions.

Elimination Problems

Medications, the illness, or the natural process of the body slowing down may affect its ability to eliminate waste products: urine and feces. A dying person may become incontinent (unable to control her bladder and/or bowels), constipated, or have diarrhea—or will sometimes experience all three at different times. It is likely previous bowel patterns will not stay the same. Changes in food and fluid intake as well as medications are all causes. Your hospice nurse will help you to prevent problems and treat them if they occur.

Toileting is viewed as a very private matter in our society. This loss of privacy can be devastating for your loved one, and there may be unpleasant sights and odors that cause deep embarrassment. Assure your loved one that it is not a problem for you. Or, if it is, try to find someone else to tend to this aspect of caregiving.

Incontinence. Incontinence is the inability to control the excretion of bodily wastes. In the United States, seven to twelve million people of all ages—including one in eight adults over age sixty-five—have bladder control problems. Although urinary incontinence can be embarrassing, bowel incontinence can be even more distressing. The loss of dignity involved, as well as the harmful effect on the skin, can be a serious problem.

Specially made underclothes, pads, and other disposable products are available if your loved one becomes incontinent. You might place a disposable cotton pad or disposable underpad beneath her. Your hospice nurse can advise you in this, and your loved one may have a preference as well.

For urinary incontinence, you might consider a catheter. Catheters drain urine into a bag so that the skin stays dry, and diapers are not necessary. For bowel incontinence, the choices are limited to a bed underpad or adult diapers. Special creams, lotions, and deodorant sprays can help clean the genital or anal area and ensure dryness afterward.

A urinal, bedpan, or commode near the bed can be of immense help. Encourage your loved one to empty her bladder and bowels often and limit fluids at night.

Diarrhea. Diarrhea is the passing of watery or loose stools three or more times a day. It may be accompanied by gas and cramping. If diarrhea occurs, contact your hospice nurse. Foods that are high in protein, calories, and potassium may help. Offer plenty of fluids, including water and clear fruit juice, and give frequent small meals rather than three substantial ones. Offer crackers, add nutmeg to food (to slow the intestines), or try the "braty" diet of bananas, rice, apple juice, dry toast, and yogurt. You might also try Kaopectate, Pepto Bismol, or Immodium A-D if your hospice nurse or physician approves.

Avoid spicy, fried, or fatty foods. Also avoid alcoholic or carbonated beverages, artificial sweeteners, very hot or very cold foods, cabbage, beans, and gum.

Constipation. Constipation is the infrequent or difficult passage of hard stools. (If your loved one hasn't had a bowel movement in three days, she is constipated.) Constipation may be uncomfortable, even painful. It may cause cramps or stomachaches. At the first sign of constipation, call your hospice nurse.

Increase high-fiber foods such as bran, wheat germ, fresh raw fruit (with skin and seeds), and fruit juice, especially prune juice. Increase activity and fluid intake, if possible. Other alternatives include laxatives, enemas, and stool softeners as prescribed by the physician. Constipation is a frequent side effect of narcotic pain medication. If your loved one is taking narcotic medications, a bowel program may be prescribed.

Your loved one should avoid extreme force or straining. She should also avoid cheese and eggs as well as over-the-counter laxatives. If your loved one seems to alternate between constipation and diarrhea, you might try Metamucil to bulk up the stool and to encourage regular bowel movements. Talk with your nurse regarding preferred methods of treatment.

Difficulty Breathing

At times, your loved one may feel like she is suffocating. Her pulse may increase, and wheezing may occur. Your loved one's breathing may become irregular and labored, and it may even stop occasionally. Be calm. If you appear alarmed, this may frighten your loved one. Instruct your loved one to do a "deep-breathing" exercise: Inhale slowly through the nose and exhale for the same amount of time through partially closed lips. Keep the mouth and lips moist. If your loved one is in bed, elevate her head and shoulders to 20 or 30 degrees by raising the head of the bed or using several pillows. Because humidity loosens phlegm, you might want to borrow, rent, or buy a humidifier or vaporizer to increase the humidity. Ask your hospice nurse if you have questions about how to keep the machine clean.

A person who has difficulty breathing feels like she is not getting enough air. Open the windows or use a fan to increase air flow through the room to help with respiratory distress. If this doesn't help, your physician may prescribe bronchodilators (medications that widen the airway) or oxygen. Delivering oxygen through small tubes inserted into the nostrils can make breathing easier. For your loved one's comfort, you might pad the part of the tube that goes over the ears with cotton or gauze held in place by adhesive tape. Because oxygen dries the mucous membranes, K-Y jelly in the nostrils may help with lubrication. Do not use any petroleum-based products. You can remove the nasal prongs every so often for five to ten minutes to give your loved one a break. Humidified oxygen is only recommended at 5 liters or higher. Oxygen is combustible, so keep it away from open flames.

If breathing becomes extremely difficult, your physician may prescribe morphine or other medications. In some cases, suctioning will keep the airway clear and prevent choking, but it is an uncomfortable procedure. Your hospice nurse will know if this is needed.

Airway Secretions

Airway secretions may cause a rattling sound in the throat. This may be more disturbing to you than to your loved one. Talk to your hospice nurse about treating these secretions with medication, although they cannot always be eliminated. Reassure your loved one that everything is all right, place her in a comfortable raised position, and provide fresh air.

Weight Loss

Your loved one may experience dramatic weight loss, and may even look emaciated or deformed. This is a natural part of the dying process. Assure your loved one that she is much more than a physical body. Discourage your loved one from staring into a mirror. She may withdraw from contact with close friends, fearing they will be dismayed at the physical deterioration. Assure your loved one that friends are coming to see her, not her body.

Fever

A fever is a temperature of more than 100.5°F orally or 101.5°F rectally (38°C and 38.6°C, respectively) that lasts for a day or more. Fever can be caused by many things. Infection, tumors, and treatments are all causes, but many people have high temperatures as the body starts to shut down. It is not uncommon for temperatures to reach 103°F at times. Your loved one might look flushed, and her head or cheeks may feel warmer than usual. Or your loved one may complain of being hot. Take her temperature to confirm that a fever exists. You might sponge the body, provide fluids often, and give acetaminophen or ibuprofen if the physician approves it. Your loved one may alternate between feeling hot and cold. Cover and uncover her body as needed. Take the temperature every four to six hours and record the result. If your loved one is chilled, lying beside her and cuddling can be beneficial for you both. Do not try to lower the fever with an ice or alcohol bath.

Seizures

Seizures are not common, but the fear of seizures is. A seizure is a sudden, involuntary, convulsive movement of the muscles. It usually lasts less than five minutes, but it may leave the person feeling confused and tired for several hours. Jerky, uncoordinated movements may indicate an oncoming seizure.

In the event of a seizure, lay the person down and turn her head to the side to keep the airway open and make vomiting easier. Your loved one may become incontinent during the seizure. Do not put anything between her teeth, as this may injure the teeth or jaw. If your loved one's bed has side rails, pad them.

Anticonvulsant medications are available, but they may cause sleepiness. Many patients prefer to remain alert despite the risk of a seizure. It's important to discuss these medications with your loved one and the hospice nurse.

Falls

Your loved one may unexpectedly drop to the floor from a standing position or from a bed, chair, wheelchair, toilet, or commode. Falls are usually caused by increasing weakness, a natural part of the dying process. Ask your loved one if she is all right. Ask about pain. Check her body for any area that looks different and might be broken. If there are no complaints of pain and nothing is out of the ordinary, help your loved one back to a seated position or back into bed. If you need help getting your loved one back to bed, call the hospice office for directions. Do not move your loved one if she complains of severe pain or has fluid draining from the mouth, nose, or ears.

To prevent falls, encourage your loved one to ask for help when getting up or walking. She should make position changes slowly and with support. Have your loved one wear nonskid socks, slippers, and shoes. Check the routes your loved one travels to make sure there is nothing she could trip over, and remove all scatter rugs.

Cognitive Impairment

Your loved one may have trouble recognizing familiar people and places, remembering past events, or thinking logically. Patients who are cognitively impaired may lose their sense of reality, become disoriented, or feel like they are going crazy. This may be due to the illness, the medication, emotional upset, or a buildup of waste products in the body.

To help your loved one, point out familiar objects. Keep a large wall calendar and large clock with a lighted face nearby. Announce the day and time first thing each morning. Circle important dates on the calendar and repeatedly remind your loved one of upcoming events. This will help give her a sense of control. You might also show photographs of people who are coming to visit or of family members she has not seen for a while.

Auditory and visual hallucinations may occur. Although not unusual, hallucinations can be very upsetting. Do not humor your loved one. Gently describe what is really happening. Explain that what she is experiencing is a result of either the illness or the medications being taken.

Agitation

Your loved one may experience restlessness, anger, fear, and anxiety, particularly in the latter part of the dying process. Agitation might result from an inability to eliminate bodily wastes. Your loved one may be worked up, wound up, uptight, and never satisfied with what you do. The question then arises, should you provide medication to relieve this agitation? Several alternatives are available: tranquilizers, pain medications, sleeping pills, or even alcohol. While any of these may reduce the agitation, all are depressants. Talk to your hospice nurse to see if these options are appropriate, and then discuss it with your loved one.

Sleep Problems

Your loved one may be afraid to go to sleep for fear of not waking up. Some terminally ill people, on the other hand, sleep more and more and eventually slip into a coma. Or, your loved one might reverse the sleep cycle, sleeping in the daytime and feeling wide awake at night. It is okay for your loved one to sleep when she feels tired, even if it is during the day.

Insomnia can be helped in a number of ways. Try to establish regular sleep patterns. You might keep a large illuminated clock by the bed and let your loved one know what time you or someone in the family will be checking on her. A bedtime routine may also help. Begin with toileting and toothbrushing, then perhaps move on to a glass of wine and a back rub. Play soft music with a slow rhythm in a quiet, dimly lit room. Keep the room well ventilated at a comfortable temperature.

Exercise and fresh air may help your loved one sleep better at night. If the insomnia is severe, talk to your hospice nurse to see whether medication might help. If your loved one is cognitively impaired, however, medication may have the opposite effect, causing agitation.

ACTIVITIES TO FILL THE DAY WITH JOY

Your loved one may attempt to withdraw, not wishing to participate in the activities you have planned. With careful guidance,
however, your loved one may come to realize how precious each
day is. See if you can interest your loved one in any of the following activities:

- Watch videos together, especially home videos.

- Watch favorite television programs together.

- Read books, magazines, or newspapers aloud.

- Listen to music and audio books.

- Go through photo albums and scrapbooks.

- Get outdoors.

- Pray or meditate together.

- Apply different lotions and creams (the sense of smell is
  among the last to go).

- Burn incense or fragrant candles.

- Have a "Happy Hour" with your loved one's favorite
  beverage and snack.

- Hold visiting hours, inviting old friends, neighbors, and
  business associates.

- Play board games and card games.

- Write thank-you notes for flowers and gifts received.

- Give a massage.

- Just talk and be close.

- Each day, try to do one thing that feels productive—and one thing for the pure joy of it.

You and your loved one can add your own activities to this list. Be sure to invite family and friends to participate.

You and your loved one may want to establish some visitor guidelines. Decide if visitors should call before coming, how long they can stay, how many visitors to have at one time, what types of activities to encourage, and the like. Some families have found it to be helpful to put a note about visiting times on the door. If visitors show up unexpectedly, always check with your loved one before showing them in. Do not assume your loved one is feeling up to a visit at that particular time.

> *We are functioning at a small fraction of our capacity to live fully [life's] total meaning of loving, caring, creating and adventuring. Consequently, the actualizing of our potential can become the most exciting adventure of our lifetime.*
>
> —Herbert Otto

EXERCISE

If your loved one is not too weak, help her exercise as much as possible. Exercise includes anything that makes a person move her muscles. Even walking to and from the bathroom is considered exercise.

If your loved one can still walk, encourage it. A cane or walker may help, or perhaps you can provide physical support. You should also encourage your loved one to sit up in a chair or wheelchair, saving the bed for naps and nighttime.

Pay special attention to range-of-motion exercises. These involve motions we use as part of our daily activities, for example, moving our head from side to side or opening and closing our hands. Your hospice nurse or physical therapist can show you how to do range-of-motion exercises.

Isometric exercises are also helpful. These exercises consist of contracting and holding a specific muscle, such as the abdominal muscle, for a count of ten. Isometric exercises can be done standing, sitting, or lying down.

Exercise releases tension, increases appetite, prevents pressure sores, promotes elimination of bodily wastes, makes a person sleep better, and improves both physical and mental health. Ideally, your loved one will be able to exercise alone (called active exercising). However, at some point, exercise may be too painful or your loved one may no longer have the energy. In this case, you may need to move your loved one's joints (called passive exercising) and change her position frequently. If your loved one does not want to be moved or is overly sensitive to touch, ask your hospice nurse or home health aide for help.

MAINTAINING SEXUALITY

A dying person's sexuality should not be denied, ignored, or discouraged. It is natural, and it need not culminate in sexual intercourse. Although this is a personal matter, sexuality should be discussed if it is an issue. In one study, over one-third of the couples continued to have sex until a few weeks before death. The entire hospice team should respect this need. The illness may cause sexual dysfunction, but that doesn't mean sexuality ceases. You can still hug and cuddle, kiss and caress. Sensual caressing and kissing can be of great comfort to your loved one and to you. Finding creative ways to express affection or sexual feelings can be fun and challenging. If sexuality issues arise, your loved one may prefer to discuss them with the hospice nurse first and then with their partner.

REDUCING STRESS

> *The last, if not the greatest, of the human freedoms: to choose their own attitude in any given circumstance.*
>
> —Bruno Bettelheim

Stress can have many negative effects on the body. It can increase muscle tension and heart rate, elevate blood pressure, cause dry mouth, and change brain waves. Both you and your loved one will undoubtedly experience stress. It is important that you learn how to reduce it. Caregivers can use all of the following techniques to reduce stress. Patients can use many of these techniques too. You might even try some of them together.

Try to keep your sense of humor. Laughing is a great stress-reducer. Also, try to remain in the present and think positively. Positive self-talk, also called affirmation, can do much to reduce stress. Tell yourself you are happy, or better yet, that you choose to be happy. Kick out negative self-talk, such as any thoughts that begin with the words "I can't . . . ."

Exercise

The physical, mental, and emotional benefits of exercise (described on page 62) are as important for caregivers as they are for patients. Make time for exercise. Consider your activity level, and don't let yourself get out of shape.

Keep a Journal

Journal writing can be very therapeutic. It offers a release, a way to transfer your problems onto paper. Never mind the spelling, grammar, or punctuation; let your thoughts and feelings flow freely. Write whatever you want, whenever you want to. Tell how your day went. Tell how you feel. Describe your fears. List the things you're thankful for. You may decide to keep writing throughout the grieving process, and perhaps throughout the rest of your life.

Use the Hospice Team

Tell members of the hospice team what you need. Let friends and family know how they can help. Don't try to go it alone.

Take Time for Yourself

Personal time-outs are important. Treat yourself to a bubble bath with your favorite music. Read a good book. Call a friend and arrange to have lunch together. Write in your journal just before bedtime. Take time to enjoy what is good about your life: your loved one's smile and touch, your brother's hug, your children's exuberance.

Find a quiet place to still your mind each day for at least twenty minutes. Try silent relaxation, chanting, visualization, or a combination.

Relaxation. Relaxation is the easiest technique. If you've never done it before, your hospice team can recommend relaxation tapes to help you get started. Find a quiet place, seat yourself comfortably, close your eyes, and try to make your mind blank. Slowly inhale through your nose to a count of eight, and then exhale through partially closed lips for a count of eight. Do this four or five times. Continue breathing, this time without counting. Try to approximate the count of eight. Do this for about ten minutes. If thoughts pop up, simply let them go and focus once again on your breathing.

Chanting. During your relaxation exercise, you might add a single word or phrase, known as a mantra. A traditional Eastern mantra is the sound "om." You might try this sound, or you can pick a sound or word of your own, such as the word love. As you practice your relaxation breathing, speak the mantra each time you exhale.

Visualization. Find a quiet room, seat yourself comfortably, close your eyes, and try to picture a favorite place. This might be a vacation spot such as a beach in Florida. Picture you and your loved one there. Smell the salty air and the suntan lotion. Hear the sea gulls' cries and the waves crashing. Feel the warm sunlight flowing into your head and then down through your neck, shoulders, chest, arms, fingers, stomach, legs, feet, and toes, relaxing each part of your body as the warmth flows through it.

Or, think of the love that you and your loved one share as a circle of light above your head. Again, feel the light enter your body and move from your head to your toes.

You might want to get a book on meditation or visualization. The benefits of these stress-reducing techniques include decreased heart rate, blood pressure, and respiration; decreased anxiety and depression; and improved sleep.

Daily caregiving is a challenge, but it is also extremely rewarding. Tending to your loved one's physical, emotional, and spiritual needs can be a wonderful experience. It is important, however, that you rely on your hospice team, and that you take care of yourself as you make this final journey with your loved one.

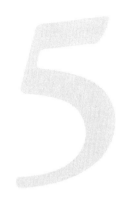

Pain: Control Is the Goal

Control of pain is really the heart of terminal care. People do not fear death so much as they fear unrelieved pain and being alone with their suffering.

—Deborah Whiting Little

John and Ella sat holding hands, discussing his pain management plan. His primary concern was to remain mentally alert, even if that meant he would experience some discomfort. The hospice team, under the direction of the nurse, had managed that beautifully. And when he did experience mild discomfort, he and Ella had a variety of techniques other than medication that worked. Hospice paid attention not only to any physical pain he experienced, but to his emotional and spiritual pain as well. He was living the final chapter of his life to the fullest.

One in three people in the United States suffer from some form of persistent or recurring pain. The costs in human suffering are incalculable. Most of us will go to great lengths to avoid pain. It is natural. If pain is severe enough and lasts long enough, it might drive a person to suicide or to request euthanasia: "I want to die—please help me." A primary goal of hospice is to eliminate such desperation brought on by pain.

Not everyone identifies with the word *pain*. Sometimes they identify better with the word *discomfort*. This discussion refers to either pain or discomfort.

Not all dying people have pain. In fact, many patients dying from cancer have no physical pain at all; a small group have mild pain; and less than half experience severe or intractable pain. However, according to Dr. Cicely Saunders, founder of the modern hospice movement: "It must not be forgotten that 'intractable' does not mean 'impossible to relieve'; its meaning is 'not easily treated.' Successful treatment may call for much imagination and persistence but pain can usually be abolished while the patient still remains alert, able to enjoy the company of those around him and often able to be up and about until his death."

Pain is more than just physical. People can experience emotional pain, spiritual pain, psychosocial pain, and financial pain. Having a team helps in many ways; hospice staff addressing concerns with the patient and family can be the best medicine.

Managing pain may be the most urgent and serious problem you and your loved one face. But it can be done. When your loved one no longer worries about pain, a great burden is lifted. He can then focus on living each day to the fullest extent possible.

UNDERSTANDING PAIN

Pain is what the person says it is.

—Margo McCaffery

The terminally ill often fear they will die an agonizing death. Pain—and fear of pain—are major challenges in hospice. Fear of pain can be as devastating as the pain itself. Understanding pain can help alleviate the fear. Also, the mere fact of confronting things one is most afraid of reduces fear and may also reduce some pain.

Pain is an unpleasant, hurtful, sometimes excruciating sensation. But it serves a purpose. Pain is our internal alarm, our natural warning system indicating that body tissues are being damaged. The sensation of pain starts when chemical substances, released when cells are injured, stimulate certain nerves. The nerves send a message up through the spinal cord to the brain to tell it that we hurt. Physicians may not be able to discover the exact cause of the pain, but it is real nonetheless.

Acute Versus Chronic Pain

Pain is either acute or chronic. *Acute pain* comes on suddenly and warns the body that you may need medical attention. A toothache, for example, sends most people off to the dentist. For your loved one, acute pain may occur with pressure ulcers or mouth sores. With effective treatment, acute pain goes away when the injury heals.

Chronic pain, on the other hand, is long-term pain caused by conditions like arthritis, heart disease, and cancer. It can last for months or years; sometimes it is permanent. Chronic pain may be caused by the pressure of a tumor, by a blockage, or by medications and other treatments. If the cause cannot be found, it can be frustrating for the patient and for those trying to manage his pain. Chronic pain may be accompanied by depression or anxiety, which may also require treatment. The best way to describe the pain is by using a specific ranking on a scale of 0-10 (ten being the most excruciating pain).

Some people talk openly of their pain. Others view pain as a sign of weakness and seek to hide it. A person's upbringing is a key factor in whether he will openly discuss physical pain. Communicate to your loved one that suffering in silence is not noble; it is unnecessary and foolish. Pain cannot be managed if it is not made known. The idea that "suffering builds character" runs counter to the hospice philosophy. Terminal pain serves no purpose and has no justification.

Also, people may fear addiction if they must have a narcotic medication. Those who need medication to help manage their pain will not become addicted. In fact, if the pain increases, the amount of medication required to help rid them of pain will also be increased. This is good pain management.

Emotional, Spiritual, and Social Pain

Pain is a complex sensation that has not only physical aspects, but emotional, spiritual, financial, and social aspects as well. A dying person may feel anxious, sad, or depressed. There may be concerns for the family and friends being left behind. There may be a fear of an afterlife, or of not having been "good enough" here on earth. There may even be financial pain as a loved one worries about how his care will be paid for, or how the family will survive the loss of his income.

Emotional pain, stress, and tension can delay or prevent the effects of pain medication and can increase the body's susceptibility to pain. A less anxious person may require smaller doses of pain medication. Encourage your loved one to talk openly about his fears.

False Beliefs about Pain

Mistaken ideas about pain can interfere with pain management. Among the false beliefs you or your loved one might hold are the following:

- Ignore pain and it will go away.

- Pain is a punishment for past wrongs.

- Pain is a way to atone for sins.

- Pain is all in the mind.

- Acknowledging pain indicates you are weak.

- Treating pain with medication may mean the medication will not work as well later when the pain is more severe.

PAIN ASSESSMENT

The intensity and frequency of pain varies according to where it is located and the individual's pain threshold. Your loved one may complain of pain. He may moan, groan, and writhe in agony. He may be restless and agitated. His heart and breathing rate may increase. If your loved one displays any of these symptoms, you need to make an assessment. (If your loved one has been in pain for a long time, these symptoms may not appear.) Ask your loved one the following questions and record the responses in your caregiver notebook:

- Where is the pain? Can you point to it? Is it deep or close to the surface?

- On a scale of zero to ten, with ten being excruciating, how intense is it?

- Is it continuous or does it come and go?

- Can you describe it? Does it throb? Ache?

- What seems to help it? To make it worse?

Note any other symptoms such as nausea, irritability, and insomnia (inability to sleep). All of this information will be important in establishing a pain management plan if one is not already in place. If you already have a pain management plan, and your loved one is still in pain, the plan should be reviewed and revised. Talk to your hospice nurse.

THE PAIN MANAGEMENT PLAN

Effective pain control is at the heart of palliative care. It includes:

- The right medications given at the right time (before pain occurs),

- Giving medication in the most effective manner (orally if possible)

- Using the least amount needed to control pain yet keep the patient lucid and coherent.

Based on what your loved one says about the level and frequency of his pain, a pain management plan will be established. This plan will vary from person to person. If no pain is the goal, the patient may be less alert. Seldom will the plan include radiation or chemotherapy. It will, however, usually include medication. It might also include other medical procedures and stress-reducing techniques that have been shown to reduce pain.

Radiation and Chemotherapy

Radiation and chemotherapy have very limited use in hospice. If a physician suggests one of these treatments, it is important that you understand the benefits and the drawbacks. The benefits of radiation and chemotherapy may include a temporary increased quality of life, better pain control, and a somewhat longer life. However, these benefits must be weighed against the drawbacks: transportation difficulties, discomfort getting to the therapy, difficulty tolerating the therapy because of weakness, and unpleasant side effects such as nausea, vomiting, diarrhea, urinary retention, and muscle twitching. A helpful question to ask is "If I have a dollar's worth of energy, how do I want to spend it?"

In most instances patients prefer other approaches to pain management.

Pain Medications

Regardless of the pain medication(s) used, a key to effective pain control is preventive scheduling.

Preventive Scheduling

Instead of treating the pain after it occurs, palliative care experts recommend *preventive scheduling:* around-the-clock pain medications administered at definite, regular intervals before the pain occurs. Preventive scheduling keeps a minimum level of pain medication in the bloodstream. Just knowing that the medication is there can greatly reduce your loved one's anxiety about pain.

The medication schedule will vary from person to person and may require some trial and error. The dosage depends on age, body size, and the level and type of pain. Most people benefit from small, steady doses of pain medication. Others need larger doses spread out over a longer period of time. Although medications may need to be given at night, waking a loved one for medication is far less disruptive than having him wake up in pain.

If the pain returns or increases, you may need to raise the dosage or increase the frequency. This is normal and is not cause for alarm. The important thing is to stay ahead of the pain.

If the schedule is working, your loved one may be tempted to stop taking the pain medication, but this is a big mistake. The pain will probably recur very soon. Write down the name of the medication, when it was given, and the dose, as it is too difficult to remember when so much is going on. Be sure to note any extra doses given and tell your hospice nurse of any changes.

Types of Pain Medications

Non-narcotic pain medications are used for mild pain. They do not require a prescription. For that reason, they are often referred to as over-the-counter or OTC drugs. The most common OTC drugs for pain are ibuprofen and acetaminophen. The usual dosage is two tablets every four to six hours. Ibuprofen should be taken with food or with antacids to prevent an upset stomach. Acetaminophen, on the other hand, should be taken on an empty stomach to improve absorption. Acetaminophen can cause liver damage in high doses. If your loved one has swallowing problems, both ibuprofen and acetaminophen are available in liquid and suppository form.

Narcotic pain medications are used for both moderate and severe pain. Most people under hospice care need narcotic pain medications at some point, either alone or with non-narcotic medications. A prescription is needed for these medications. The most commonly prescribed narcotic is long-acting morphine. Morphine is available in controlled-release tablets for prolonged pain relief.

Other narcotic pain medications include codeine, hydromorphone (brand name Dilaudid), levorphanol, methadone (Dolophine), oxycodone (Percodan or Percocet), and hydrocodone (Vicodin).

Other medications may be used along with narcotics to enhance their effectiveness. These are called *co-analgesics*. They may include nonsteroidal anti-inflammatory drugs (NSAIDs), antidepressants, anticonvulsants, muscle relaxants, corticosteroids, and tranquilizers such as Valium. Other medications reduce neuropathic pain and also manage constipation, which is a common side effect of narcotic medication.

Administering Pain Medications

Pain medications can be administered in many ways. The first choice is orally (by mouth) in the form of pills, tablets, capsules, or liquids. This is the simplest and least invasive approach for your loved one. If medications are administered orally but your loved one refuses to take them and is cognitively impaired, he may not realize the implications: The pain will return. If you believe your loved one would take them if he was thinking clearly, you might try to disguise the medications by grinding them up and putting them in food or beverages. This can be a difficult decision.

If your loved one has difficulty swallowing or is vomiting frequently, you may need to explore other alternatives. Often medications are effectively administered sublingually (under the tongue). These are absorbed very quickly. Other medications are administered transdermally (through a skin patch). Transdermal medications are absorbed slowly through the skin over the course of three days. They take eighteen hours to reach their full effect. That is why this route of delivery may be a problem. Rectal suppositories may also be used. Hospice nurses can teach caregivers how to insert rectal medications effectively and with dignity.

If medications must be given continuously, they may be administered intravenously (directly into the vein) or intrathecally (directly into the spinal cord). For people requiring high doses of a narcotic, a continuous-drip infusion pump may be used to release the narcotic into the body at a constant rate. The pump can be worn on the body, and patients can give themselves "bolus" or additional doses if needed. The pump is designed so patients cannot overdose. The hospice nurse and pharmacist can be very helpful.

Other medications are injected subcutaneously (under the skin), particularly if the patient has collapsed veins or is emaciated. These medications may also be given continuously by infusion pump. Medications may also be given intramuscularly (injected into the muscle) but this is rare.

Occasionally, pain medications are administered through a nebulizer machine. In these cases, the patient inhales the medication through a mask or mouthpiece.

If medications must be injected, the hospice nurse will train you. Injecting medications may sound difficult or frightening at first, but it is really quite simple once you learn how.

Side Effects

Constipation is one of the most common side effects of morphine and other narcotic pain medications. Your loved one will require a laxative. The hospice nurse will recommend a bowel program. Senekot, made from vegetables, is usually recommended for constipation. It is available over the counter. It is very important to follow this program, especially if the patient has never before had a problem with being constipated. It is essential to take it consistently to avoid the side effects of constipation.

Nausea is common, although it will often go away after a few days. The hospice physician may prescribe medication to control nausea.

Sleepiness is another frequent side effect. In fact, the word narcotic means "sleep inducing." Narcotics may seem to cause sedation during the first few days, but the patient may simply be catching up on lost sleep or finally sleeping without worry of the pain coming back.

Mental confusion is a less common side effect. Confusion may occur when a new narcotic is started or increased. This may be temporary. It may also occur as the patient begins to decline.

Practical Matters

Ask your hospice physician or nurse about all medications prescribed and their side effects. Some of these medications are potent chemicals, and you need to know why they have been prescribed and what they are expected to do.

- Write down the names of all the medications, getting the correct spellings.

- Find out if specific brand names are being prescribed or if the pharmacist can choose a generic drug.

- If you have any questions about the possible side effects, ask.

- Never use pain medication to control your loved one's behavior.

- Keep at least one week's supply of all medications on hand. You don't want to run out. Some medications need a signed physician prescription each time they are refilled. Allow more time for these.

- Keep all medications out of the reach of children.

- Your hospice program may provide you with a "comfort kit" of special medications to be used in the event your loved one has some specific symptoms. Keep them safe but handy, and let your hospice nurse know where they are kept so they can be found and used quickly, if needed.

When Patients Refuse to Take Their Medication

If your loved one refuses to take his pain medication, the pain will return. It is important to find out why your loved one is refusing the medication. He may have a number of fears that, when not addressed, could become significant barriers to pain management.

Fear of building up a tolerance. Some patients worry that taking medication for moderate pain will leave them with no recourse if their pain later becomes severe. One grandmother prided herself on taking a minimum amount of medication, breaking her aspirins in half because "You never know when you might really need them." If your loved one is worried about building up a tolerance, explain that there is no such thing as a maximum dose. If the pain increases, the hospice physician will increase the dose as often as needed.

Fear of an overdose. It is difficult to overdose on narcotics if they are taken routinely. Signs of overdose include drowsiness, a thick tongue, hallucinations, confusion, slurred speech, and slowed breathing (ten breaths or fewer in one minute). If these symptoms occur, call your hospice nurse or physician. If your loved one has had pain for a long time and has just begun taking a narcotic, he may feel extremely drowsy. This is not an overdose. Drowsiness is a natural side effect of the medication and may resolve within 72 hours, or it could be a sign of approaching death.

Fear of addiction. Most research shows that people who use narcotics to relieve pain do not become addicted. Hospice patients use narcotics for pain relief, not for emotional or psychological relief. Addiction occurs when there is no pain in the body for the medication to work on. Patients with long-term severe pain may become dependent on their medication, but this is not drug abuse. A person dependent upon pain medication is no more an "addict" than a diabetic dependent on insulin. If the pain lessens after some form of treatment, the dosage may be decreased.

Nonpharmaceutical Treatment of Pain

> *A couple of times a day I sit quietly and visualize my body fighting the AIDS virus. It's the same as me sitting and seeing myself hit the perfect serve. I did that often when I was an athlete.*
>
> —**Arthur Ashe, tennis player who died of AIDS**

Pain management does not rely solely on the use of medications. A number of nonpharmaceutical options exist to help control pain. These can be used alone or in conjunction with pain medication.

Reducing Pain by Reducing Stress and Tension

Perhaps no human experience is more stressful than dying. Dying brings an inevitable sense of loss and grief, even before the actual death occurs. This stress can intensify pain, causing even more stress. Pain and stress feed off one another. Muscular pain and painful breathing make a person tense up even more, and this, too, can make the pain worse. To break the cycle, try to reduce your loved one's stress.

Isometric exercises can help relax the muscles. Have your loved one begin by tensing his facial muscles, holding them for ten seconds, and then releasing them. Do the same thing with the neck muscles. Continue down through the body: shoulders, arms, hands, stomach, buttocks, thighs, calves, and feet.

A gentle massage might help relax your loved one's muscles. You might want to use a non-alcohol-based lotion. If you use scented lotion, be sure the scent is pleasing to him. During the massage, you and your loved one might practice deep-breathing exercises. A foot massage is almost always a pleasure.

Visualization is a process of imagining scenes that make a person happy or help resolve problems. Talking your loved one through positive images or memories can help divert the pain. A classic example: When a cancer patient imagines his white blood cells attacking and destroying the cancer, the patient may begin to relax—and his pain will often decrease.

Heat therapy is yet another option. To relax the muscles, apply a hot-water bottle or heating pad. A warm bath might also be soothing. Avoid hot water, as this can dry the skin, and line the bathtub with towels to provide a cushion. Devices are available to turn a regular bathtub into a Jacuzzi. Although heat therapy can be beneficial, always consider the effort and/or pain involved in getting in and out of the tub.

Cold therapy can be used to relax muscles by slowing circulation. Place a piece of ice in a towel and rub it slowly over the painful area for about ten minutes. Your hospice nurse can demonstrate this technique and advise you of precautions. Do not use this approach if your loved one's pain is caused by poor circulation.

Music is another way to relax. Terminal illness usually does not affect one's hearing. Music can provide a soothing distraction and give your loved one pleasure, especially if someone else is there to share the experience.

Distractions have been found to raise pain threshold by as much as 45 percent. Work puzzles together. Play "Do you remember when?" Hold hands and share your happy memories. Watch old slapstick movies together and laugh. Sexual relations can also reduce stress and pain. Finally, think positively. Concentrate on what your loved one can still do. The power of positive thinking is tremendous.

Other Approaches to Controlling Pain

Other options for controlling pain include electrical stimulation (TENS or Transcutaneous Electrical Nerve Stimulation), hypnosis, biofeedback, and acupuncture. In specific circumstances, palliative surgery, such as a cordotomy or nerve block, can give dramatic relief. Your hospice nurse or physician can explain these options if you and your loved one are interested.

Cutting down on stimulants such as the caffeine in coffee, tea, and some soft drinks may also reduce your loved one's pain

The key player in managing pain is your loved one. If he speaks of pain, it is real, even if the cause of the pain cannot be established. Pain management is one of the most challenging aspects of caregiving. Reach out to your hospice team for help. You can rely on their expertise.

Find out if there is a pain management center, a palliative care center, or a support group in your area. Your loved one's pain can be managed.

Allied Therapies:
Creating Wholeness and Meaning

Every person is a complex and beautiful whole, with many dimensions. Every one of those dimensions— physical, psychological, social, cultural, spiritual—is related to our health and well-being.

—Becky Myrick, holistic health practitioner

The day that Ella and John decided to get married, they had gone to the movie Breakfast at Tiffanys. *The signature song "Moon River" became their special song from that day forward, and it brought back happy memories whenever they heard it. During their visit with the hospice music therapist, they asked her to sing "Moon River," and became tearful as they listened. They talked about their fears and sadness at being separated after almost 50 years of marriage. They expressed appreciation for the happiness each had brought to the other. The words of the song, which evoke images of crossing the river, being a dream maker and a heart breaker, provided a rich opportunity to talk about their beliefs about life and death, grief and gratitude. After this serious but sweet conversation, they asked the music therapist to sing other songs—from their courtship years, their trip to Norway, and songs their children used to love—as they remembered and celebrated the good times they had together.*

HOLISTIC PHILOSOPHY OF CARE

Beyond just healing or helping the physical body, holistic practice means helping people see themselves with new eyes, as whole human beings. Hospice, though a part of traditional western medical care, has always taken a holistic approach to treating patients, that is, taking into account the mind and spirit as well as the body in their approach to caring for the hospice patient. Increasingly, our traditional medical system is also moving in this direction.

Allied or complementary therapies are practices from traditions other than western medicine such as massage, acupuncture, or music therapy that may be part of holistic care. The terms *complementary* or *allied* stem from the idea that these methods should not replace but rather work with traditional medical treatment. Intrinsic to the process of healing is a true partnership between practitioner and patient. It is no surprise then that allied therapies are a welcome addition to many hospice programs. Allied therapists use nondrug interventions to enhance one's sense of well-being, reduce stress, and promote healing.

All human beings hold a set of assumptions about their sense of self-worth and purpose within a world that is good and meaningful. A traumatic life event can change these assumptions dramatically. Individuals experiencing significant loss or change very often express a need to re-create meaning in order to heal.

When holistic practitioners talk about healing, they are not necessarily talking about curing. Curing is the elimination of disease. Healing is always optimistic or hopeful, and involves the creation of new meaning in one's life. Healing is always possible, while curing may not be.

Perhaps the most important aspect of holistic health is learning to manage stress. Managing stress often requires changes in lifestyle and self-awareness. It may mean recognizing the mind-body connection, knowing how to use the relaxation response, taking care of your body, and building a supportive network. Reducing stress often decreases negative mood states; it can improve one's thinking and ability to concentrate or find healing.

Questions about Allied Therapy in Hospice

Do all programs offer allied therapies?

Not all do. An increasing number of hospice programs, however, have complementary therapists on staff, usually music therapists art therapists, and massage therapists who work as part of the hospice team. This chapter addresses music therapy and massage therapy. Other types of holistic therapies include art, poetry, horticulture, movement, pet, or aromatherapies. Some programs offer healing touch or other somatic approaches.

Who pays for allied therapies?

Complementary therapies are not covered as part of the Medicare hospice benefit or by private insurance. When allied therapists are part of a hospice program, they are usually supported by a foundation or through donations and memorial bequests.

Are allied therapies a good fit for my loved one?

You may want to talk to your hospice nurse about whether complementary therapies fit the needs of your loved one. Many patients and their families request music or massage therapy when they first enter the hospice program. Some receive these therapies for a specific need for only a few sessions. Others consider allied therapies a central part of ongoing hospice care.

MUSIC THERAPY

> *The music therapist in hospice care . . . has to search for the thread of music in the life of each person and in this process discover where it wove itself into meaning for that individual*
>
> – Susan Munro, *Music Therapy in Palliative/Hospice Care*

Music is an important part of who we are as human beings, so it is no surprise that it remains important at the end of our lives. Because music affects all parts of our selves—the physical, emotional, psychological, and spiritual—music therapy is by its nature holistic. Music therapists are trained to use the healing benefits of music in a wide variety of ways. Each music therapy session is tailored to the particular needs and situation of your loved one.

Music, either alone or with guided imagery, can reduce the perception of pain by evoking the relaxation response. Music therapists can help your loved one relax through rhythmic entrainment. Rhythmic entrainment means falling naturally into the same rhythmic pattern as the music being played or sung; it is a gradual process led by the music therapist. Deep breathing is another important part of relaxation. If your loved one sings, breathing naturally deepens. If your loved one does not sing, breathing will still deepen as she entrains to the rhythm chosen by the music therapist.

Underlying emotional or spiritual pain can sometimes increase the perception of physical pain. Due to the close link between memory, emotion, and music, music therapy can be very effective in helping you and your loved one address emotional or spiritual issues. Music can help us remember times when we felt happy or times that were difficult and need resolution. Music helps us express our emotions and to resolve them. Music commonly evokes tears but also laughter and joy. A skilled music therapist can help your loved one discover new ways of looking at and thinking about her life, illness, or imminent death.

Music is essential to most people's spiritual or religious life. Music can be especially comforting if your loved one can no longer attend his place of worship. The music therapist can help provide your loved one with music to soothe the spirit, whether it is traditional religious music or music that evokes an aesthetically pleasing or transcendent experience. A music therapist can help the patient or family members to plan a memorial service or celebrate a special occasion such as a birthday or an anniversary.

Music therapy can address a patient's diminished ability to understand or reason due to illness or injury. The rhythm and structure of music often helps patients become more alert and responsive, especially when dementia or brain injury exists. Improved alertness helps your loved one enjoy her final days, and increases the quality of time spent with family and friends. When speech has become difficult or impossible, music therapy can create another means of communication. If your loved one has a personal association with particular songs or music styles, listening to that music can evoke powerful memories and offer messages to patients who may have lost their normal ability to interact.

Music therapy may have the following healing effects. It may

- Reduce anxiety.

- Induce the relaxation response.

- Help your loved one to express emotions.

- Strengthen family and social relationships.

- Lead your loved one to reflect on the meaning of her life.

- Provide social and emotional support.

- Reduce stress.

- Improve verbal or cognitive functioning.

- Improve your loved one's level of alertness.

- Provide spiritual comfort.

- Inspire a transcendent or spiritual experience.

- Inspire the family to plan music for the memorial service or funeral.

- Reduce your loved one's perception of pain or nausea.

- Evoke memories.

- Create joyful or meaningful experiences.

- Assist your loved one with legacy projects such as writing a song.

Common Questions about Music Therapy

What happens in a typical music therapy session?

No two music therapy sessions are alike. On the first visit, the music therapist will assess your loved one's emotional and cognitive status, support system, pain, and religious or spiritual associations. The therapist will also discuss your loved one's preferences for different types of music and favorite or special songs. During the assessment, the music therapist will plan the possible uses of music therapy with you and your loved one.

The music therapist will follow up with visits that may occur weekly, several times a month, or just once or twice. During regular visits, the therapist will use a variety of instruments or music, depending upon individual needs. This may include recorded music, but most often the music therapist will play live music. On occasion, your loved one, too, may play music or sing.

Why do I need a music therapist when I have a CD collection?

Music therapy is much more than simply listening to recorded music. Although recorded music can be helpful at certain times, working with a trained music therapist can lead to much deeper and richer uses of music.

My loved one can no longer respond. Will she benefit from music therapy?

Hearing is believed to be the last sense to leave us before we die. Music can be comforting and calming, not only for the patient but also for caregivers who may be exhausted, scared, or angry. Occasionally a dying patient who has not responded to verbal interaction does respond to music with a smile, tapping a toe, or reaching out with a hand. If you have been working with a music therapist already, remember that the music therapist will adjust the music therapy session to fit your loved one's current condition.

MASSAGE THERAPY

*Human touch can communicate the energy
of life itself.*

—William Frick

Human touch is essential to normal development and even to survival. It is also essential for the body-mind-spirit to work together effectively. Massage therapy can assist hospice patients by bringing relaxation and relief of pain, anxiety, depression, and restlessness. It can also help overcome nausea from chemotherapy and reduce overall aches and muscle pain and feelings of isolation. Massage therapy increasingly is used for reduction of swelling (edema) through the use of lymphatic drainage massage, in which the lymph fluids are moved back to the lymph node areas for reprocessing. Patients can then be more active and mobile with less discomfort overall and less irritation to the skin.

Soft tissue manipulation (massage) does not spread cancer. In fact, cancer patients are finding massage relieves symptoms. A large study of over 1,200 cancer patients who received massage therapy, performed at the Memorial Sloan-Kettering Cancer Center in New York (2001–2004), demonstrated that pain-symptom scores were reduced by approximately 50 percent, even for patients who reported high levels of pain initially. Benefits persisted particularly for outpatients, with no evidence of a return to previous levels of pain.

Cancer pain is affected by a variety of influences, including fear, loneliness, memories, and beliefs as well as physiological reasons. One of the greatest current challenges in medicine is dealing with the pain that accompanies metastasized cancer. Because pain comes from a multitude of influences, the best pain management uses a multi-modal approach, a combination of drug and non-drug interventions. When patients have a variety of ways to reduce pain, they perceive pain to be less intense. Guided imagery accompanied by relaxation can also be very helpful in overcoming pain of all kinds.

What to Expect from the Hospice Massage Therapist

The therapist will adapt the massage according to the needs of your loved one, often applying gentle touch through Swedish massage, pressure points, reflexology, or other forms of therapeutic touch. The therapist can adjust your loved one's body position so that she is comfortable. In most cases, the therapist will not ask a patient to lie on her stomach, as this may be uncomfortable. Your loved one's back is usually massaged while lying on her side in bed. The therapist will be sensitive to modesty concerns through proper draping with sheets or blankets.

In many cases, the therapist will gladly teach simple massage techniques to family members or caregivers. This can be especially helpful for patients with swelling. It also gives family members something beneficial to do for their loved one, and a way to communicate through touch.

A True Story

Joe was a patient in hospice who had lived with leg pain for many years. His diagnosis was kidney failure but no one knew why he had such terrible leg pain. He had gone to a highly regarded clinic where they gave him many kinds of medication for more than ten years, but nothing helped the leg pain. Within the hospice plan, Joe received a combination of deep tissue, Swedish, and sports massage on his legs. Joe reported that no one at any of the other clinics had ever touched his legs, even though that was where his pain resided. After the first massage therapy visit, his leg pain was gone with no return during his remaining months of life.

Quality of life is a central issue for hospice patients. They must struggle to perform daily functions while dealing with pain, weakness, and fatigue. Depression can result and families can become overwhelmed trying to encourage their loved ones. Depression or apathy can lead to a downward spiral in the disease process, as emotions can directly affect the immune system. Massage brings relief from depression and fatigue, renewing energy and wholeness of self. It can also be a catalyst for emotional expression and psychological release.

Common Questions about Massage Therapy

Will the therapist be working with a massage table?
Not usually. Most patients are not able to get on and off a table. So, most often the therapist will work with patients in their beds. Hospital beds work well but are not necessary. Couches are usually too low for the massage therapist to work safely and effectively. Massage therapy can also be given with the patient sitting in a chair.

Will the patient need to remove clothing (and thereby get cold)?
The patient and the therapist can decide what clothing needs to be removed, depending on the type of massage. When clothing is removed, a sheet or blanket is always used to cover the areas of the body that are not being massaged at the moment. Often patients discover a massage makes them warmer because it helps increase circulation very rapidly. This is a pleasant sensation for most patients. The therapist will add extra blankets if needed.

What kind of massage will the patient receive?
Your loved one's massage therapist has probably trained in a variety of techniques. Some examples are Swedish, Esalen, reflexology, pressure points, lymphatic relief, energy work, and more. Some people prefer light touch, while others prefer deep pressure. Please communicate your loved one's preferences to the massage therapist.

Will you use lotion?
Many therapists use lotions that are light and nongreasy. If your loved one prefers another lotion, you should tell your massage therapist.

How long do visits last and how often do they occur?
The therapist and the healthcare team will plan visits based upon individual needs. Visits usually last one hour or less. Typically, visits occur more often when there is pain, swelling, or anxiety. If regular visits are indicated, they might take place anywhere from once a week to once a month.

HOLISTIC CARE AT THE END OF LIFE

A True Story

Jack, a hospice patient at an assisted living facility, had been very skeptical about using massage therapy. Being a very modest and private man, he was reluctant to let anyone touch him. Since he had pain and stiffness in his back, his nurse encouraged him to try massage therapy. Once he tried it, he enjoyed it and it gave him great relief.

Jack had been just as skeptical of music therapy. His family knew how much he loved music and how he had enjoyed dancing with his beloved wife when she was alive, so they encouraged him to try it. During the first visit Jack said to the music therapist, "Now I understand this music therapy. When you bring back the good memories, you bring the good feelings that go with it."

Several times Jack requested that both therapists visit at the same time. As he listened to music from his past and received massage on his back, Jack would sometimes cry, sometimes laugh. Often he would state, "I can't believe I waited until I was almost 90 years old to have one of these things. The people in the dining room always know when I've had my music and massage therapy. They tell me I float into the dining room."

Allied therapies can improve the quality of your loved one's life in ways you may not expect. Although holistic approaches may not be right for everyone, they bring wholeness, meaning, and healing to many hospice patients. Talk with your hospice nurse about whether your program offers music therapy, massage therapy, or one of many other allied therapies. Your hospice nurse can help you decide what is best for you and your loved one.

7

Nutrition: Nourishment Is More Than Food and Drink

Dealing with a loved one who doesn't eat or eats
very little is part of the process of letting go.

—Deborah Duda

One morning, Ella sat with Jennifer, the hospice nurse, and shared her frustration: "John's eating less and less each day. He used to have such a big appetite, but now he can barely finish a bowl of soup. I fix his favorite dishes, and he says he doesn't feel like eating. How's he supposed to keep up his strength?"

"Ella," Jennifer responded, placing her hand gently on Ella's, "This is to be expected and accepted as part of the dying process. Let's not force it. It's not our failure. John will eat and drink when he needs to and wants to."

Food not only provides energy and sustains strength, it is an important part of all cultures. In many cultures sharing food is the highest form of showing love. Food is at the center of most holidays and special occasions—the Thanksgiving turkey, a favorite kind of birthday cake, a special restaurant on anniversaries. Food is socially significant.

We also know that we must eat to live. When a loved one's eating decreases greatly or stops entirely, it forces us to confront the reality that our loved one is not going to get better.

As the end of life approaches, it is normal to lose the desire for food and fluids. The body knows what it needs and will begin to conserve the energy it normally spends on eating. Spiritual energy rather than physical strength will sustain your loved one from here on.

It can be distressing when a loved one does not eat. Your inability to nourish your loved one may, in fact, be one of the most frustrating and upsetting aspects of caregiving. Try to accept it as an expected, normal part of the dying process. Pressuring your loved one to eat will only heighten frustrations. Comments like, "Please, just try a little of this" and "You're not eating enough" become irritating to someone who simply has no appetite.

Let your loved one choose whether or not to eat. Pay close attention to his preferences, and make meals as relaxing and comfortable as possible. This will be far more satisfying than an eating routine that no longer provides the energy, comfort, or pleasure it once did.

It is normal to fear what will happen if your loved one doesn't eat. Although suffering may seem inevitable, dying patients generally do *not* experience hunger or discomfort. If they are hungry, most are satisfied with small amounts of food. In the last days, forgoing food and drink actually eases death. It lessens consciousness, promotes sleep, and diminishes pain.

LOSS OF APPETITE

> *Recognize that loss of appetite is a real loss for*
> *everyone, like all losses that are a part of illness.*
>
> —Deborah Duda

Hospice patients lose their appetite or eat less than normal for a variety of reasons. As bodily functions gradually slow and then cease, what little energy remains is directed toward maintaining the vital functions of the heart, lungs, and brain. This is part of the body's natural preparation to stop functioning altogether. In addition, illness often changes how foods taste or smell. Favorite meals may no longer hold the same appeal.

When cancer cells are present, certain chemicals are released that affect the brain's appetite center. This may also affect the taste buds, making food taste different. Chemotherapy, radiation therapy, and some medications may also contribute to loss of appetite.

Sometimes, nausea or swallowing difficulties reduce a person's desire to eat. Pain, fatigue, stress, depression, tumor growth, or fear of impending death may affect appetite as well. Constipation or diarrhea could become issues. Like other aspects of hospice care, when it comes to eating and drinking, *comfort* is the focus.

MAKING MEALTIMES ENJOYABLE

Although eating and drinking may not be as important physically, meals and snacks can still bring your loved one pleasure. Some of the following suggestions may work:

- Forget "good" nutrition. Let your loved one decide what and how much to eat.

- Offer choices, but do not prod.

- Plan small, frequent meals with favorite foods.

- Serve meals when your loved one is rested and appears comfortable.

- To stimulate appetite, encourage your loved one to do range-of-motion exercises, actively or passively, one hour before mealtime.

- Try to eliminate cooking odors by serving food cold or at room temperature. The smell of food can precipitate nausea or make a person feel full.

- Adjust the seasonings in food to accommodate taste changes. Basil, oregano, tarragon, and lemon are usually well tolerated.

- Add a high-protein supplement to the meal such as Ensure, Isocal, or Citrotein. Other sources of protein include soy products, chicken, fish, turkey, eggs, and some dairy products.

- Concentrate on high-calorie foods. Protein supplements can add 350 calories a day.

- Keep portions small.

- Serve beverages between meals rather than with meals. Liquids at mealtime can make your loved one feel full.

- Set an attractive tray or table in an airy, cheerful environment.

- Encourage your loved one to eat with the family for as long as possible.

- Make the most of breakfast time. Appetite tends to decrease as the day goes on.

- Create a relaxed, unhurried mealtime by eating together or watching a favorite television program while eating.

- Eat the same thing as your loved one.

- Don't let mealtime become a battleground. Do not nag.

- Encourage your loved one to feed himself for as long as possible.

- If your loved one doesn't want to eat, do not view this as your failure.

- Allow your loved one to rest after meals, but keep the head of the bed elevated to promote digestion.

FLUID NEEDS

Liquids keep the skin and mucous membranes moist, and they aid the removal of bodily wastes. Nonetheless, if your loved one refuses liquids, don't force it. At this point, dehydration causes no discomfort. In fact, it is more peaceful to decline in a state of dehydration than fluid overload.

It is best to serve beverages between meals. Liquids at mealtime can make your loved one feel too full to eat. Also, encourage your loved one to drink quality liquids. High-calorie, high-protein drinks, for example, provide both fluids and nutrition (Instant Breakfast, Ensure, Boost). You can fortify milk by adding nonfat dry milk to whole milk. (For better flavor, refrigerate the mixture at least four hours before drinking.) Foods such as Jell-O, pudding, ice cream, yogurt, milkshakes, and eggnog are a good source of fluids. If your loved one has trouble with dairy products, try crushing Popsicles or frozen fruit juice from an ice cube tray.

COMMON CAUSES OF EATING PROBLEMS

Swallowing difficulties, mouth sores, nausea, or other conditions may hamper your loved one's desire for food. There are ways to overcome these. If you have questions or concerns, talk with your hospice nurse. The nurse might have you consult a dietitian. If your loved one is having symptoms such as dry mouth or mouth sores, your hospice physician might work with you, the nurse, and your loved one to control these symptoms.

Dry Mouth
Mouth dryness, or xerostomia, is a common problem for many ill people. Certain medications, breathing through the mouth, breathing dehumidified oxygen, and general dehydration can all slow saliva production. To relieve dry mouth, some of the following suggestions may help:

- Use an artificial saliva preparation, mouth-coating spray, or wetting agent.

- Rinse the mouth every two hours with a lubricant. One option is a mixture of 1 teaspoon salt to 1 quart warm water. Another option is to add 1/4 teaspoon glycerin to 1 cup water. You may swish and spit but do not swallow the mixture.

- Moisten foods with sauces, gravies, yogurt, or salad dressing.

- Offer frequent sips of liquid, small chips of ice, frozen pieces of fruit or fruit juice, or Popsicles to suck on. Frozen grapes or watermelon are popular.

- Use a moisturizer on the lips.

- Offer sugar-free gum or candy. Lemon drops and other citrus-flavored candies work well.

- Keep a water bottle near your loved one.

- Avoid serving foods that require a lot of chewing.

Mouth Sores

The linings of the mouth and throat are among the most sensitive areas of the body. Mouth sores are common after chemotherapy but are also caused by radiation therapy, infection, dehydration, poor mouth care, oxygen therapy, alcohol, tobacco, or lack of protein. Mouth sores can make eating painful. They're like having little cuts or ulcers in the mouth. The sores, which can bleed, may be very red or have small white patches in the middle.

The key to healing or avoiding mouth sores is to clean the mouth at least twice a day. Gently brush the teeth and gums with a soft, nylon-bristle toothbrush. To soften the bristles even more, soak the brush in hot water before and during brushing. If the toothbrush hurts, use a cotton swab, a Popsicle stick wrapped in gauze, or a toothette. (A toothette is a small sponge specially designed for oral care and often used in hospitals. *A toothette should not be used if the mouth is ulcerated.* Instead, use a cotton swab dipped in cold water.) Use a nonabrasive toothpaste or a baking soda solution. Rinse the toothbrush well after each use and store it in a cool, dry place. If your loved one wears dentures, remove and clean the dentures between meals. Dentures should *not* be worn if your loved one has severe mouth sores.

Some of the following suggestions may also help prevent or relieve mouth sores:

- Ask your hospice physician for a prescription to numb the mouth and treat the sores.

- Gently rinse the mouth before and after meals and at bedtime with a solution of 1 teaspoon baking soda in 1 cup warm water.

- Avoid mouthwashes that contain large amounts of salt, alcohol, or other irritants.

- Apply moisturizer to the lips and corners of the mouth to prevent cracking.

- Make foods soft and moist. If necessary, puree them.

- Offer cool foods or beverages.

- Provide ice chips or frozen pieces of fruit to suck on.

Swallowing Difficulties

Your loved one may gag, cough, spit, or complain of pain when trying to swallow. Swallowing difficulties are a common side effect of chemotherapy or radiation therapy to the throat or chest area. They are often caused by dry mouth, mouth sores, a tumor, or treatable infections such as thrush. The following suggestions might make swallowing more comfortable:

- Provide a local anesthetic or pain reliever, such as viscous lidocaine (available by prescription) or liquid Tylenol.

- Offer bland foods that are soft, smooth, and high in calories and protein such as yogurt, milk shakes, or puddings.

- Add sauces and gravies to dry food.

- Avoid serving hard or sticky foods. Mash foods to baby-food consistency.

- Offer liquids that have some consistency, such as milk shakes or blenderized fruit. These are easier to swallow than clear liquids.

- Freeze soft and liquid foods onto a stick and feed slowly.

- Have your loved one eat while sitting upright. If your loved one is bedridden, get as close to a sitting position as he can manage.

- Provide a straw for liquids and soft foods.

- Encourage your loved one to take a deep breath before swallowing and to exhale or cough after each bite.

Do not force fluids if your loved one coughs soon after drinking—swallowing reflexes may be sluggish. The body lets us know when it no longer desires or can tolerate food or liquids. The loss of this desire is a signal that the body is making itself ready to die. As weakness increases, it will be more difficult for your loved one to swallow. If you notice food is accumulating in your loved one's cheeks, do not continue to feed him.

Taste Changes

To your loved one, the taste of food may change from day to day. He may complain that foods taste "off," metallic, or too sweet. On some days, food may have lost its taste entirely. Ask your loved one what tastes best and what doesn't taste good. Respect these preferences and be flexible. Remember that the goal is to make eating an enjoyable experience. If food just doesn't taste the same, the following suggestions may help:

- Experiment with herbs and spices. Your loved one may like spicier foods at this time.

- Serve food cold or at room temperature. Many foods, including meat and poultry, taste better when they are not hot.

- Serve sorbet, sherbet, and fruit smoothies.

- Serve eggs, which often taste good when meat does not.

- Rinse your loved one's mouth with fruit juice, wine, tea, ginger ale, club soda, or salted water before eating. This helps clear the taste buds.

Nausea or Vomiting

Sometimes, offensive tastes or smells are so powerful that patients become nauseated. Anxiety, a new drug, and constipation could play a part in nausea as well.

Nausea and vomiting make eating and drinking nearly impossible. Fortunately, there are several medications that can help a queasy stomach. If nausea or vomiting occur, it's important to tell your hospice nurse. The following suggestions may also bring relief:

- Administer nausea or pain medications an hour before eating.

- Offer small meals throughout the day if the nausea occurs only between meals.

- Offer mildly seasoned foods and avoid sweet, spicy, fatty, or greasy foods.

- Offer plain foods that are broiled, boiled, steamed, or baked.

- Provide dry foods, such as crackers, first thing in the morning.

- Serve food cold or at room temperature to decrease its smell and taste.

- Offer cool, clear beverages such as ginger ale, apple juice, and broth.

- Provide a distraction while your loved one eats. Turn on music or watch a television program together. Your loved one may prefer not to talk—the effort may make the nausea worse.

- Use aromatic scents along with relaxation techniques at the first sign of nausea.

- After your loved one has eaten, encourage him to rest by sitting up or reclining with his head and shoulders elevated. Your loved one should not lie flat for at least two hours after eating.

- Keep a record of when, how often and how much your loved one vomits.

Nausea accompanied by vomiting can be a serious problem. Your loved one may lose important medications as well as vital fluids. Clean up the vomit quickly; otherwise the smell may bring on more vomiting. Ventilate the room and offer to rinse your loved one's mouth and brush his teeth to remove the taste. A mouthwash might also be appreciated.

Constipation

Constipation is a common problem for people with advanced illnesses. Pain medications are often the main cause; however, pain, lack of activity, a low-fiber diet, poor fluid intake, and general weakness can contribute to constipation as well. Generally, your loved one should have at least one bowel movement every three days, even if not eating, and the stool should not be so hard it is difficult to pass.

Because constipation can cause stomachaches, cramps, and general discomfort, your hospice physician may prescribe a laxative, stool softener, and/or suppository. The following suggestions may also help:

- Add prunes and prune juice to the diet.

- Avoid foods that can cause constipation, such as cheese and eggs.

- Offer fiber-rich foods such as fruits, nuts, whole grains, and popcorn.

- Provide plenty of liquids. Hot liquids stimulate bowel activity. A cup of tea or warm water with lemon, taken first thing in the morning, can act as a gentle, natural laxative.

- Increase daily activity if possible.

- Do not provide over-the-counter laxatives unless prescribed by the doctor.

- Have your loved one take any prescribed stool softener on a regular schedule.

- Encourage your loved one to use the toilet or commode, if possible, instead of a bedpan.

Diarrhea

Diarrhea is loose or watery stools passed three or more times a day. Causes include drug reactions, infection, anxiety, food sensitivity, and injury to the intestinal tract. Unless diarrhea continues for several days, or your loved one is getting weak from dehydration, it's often best to let it run its course.

Be sure that your loved one is cleaned well after each bowel movement. You might apply a soothing cream to the anal area or use a prescription anesthetic ointment. Your hospice doctor may prescribe an antidiarrheal drug. To help control diarrhea through nutrition, encourage your loved one to

- Eat foods high in protein, calories, and potassium but low in fiber. Try cottage cheese, eggs, boiled white rice, cooked cereals, and bananas.

- Choose breads, cereals, and pasta made with white flour.

- Eat fewer fruits and vegetables and drink clear fruit juices.

- Drink fluids at room temperature. Hot or cold liquids may stimulate bowel movements. Avoid caffeinated beverages.

ARTIFICIAL HYDRATION
AND NUTRITION

When a dying patient can no longer take in food or fluid by mouth, artificial feeding tubes or IV needles can deliver fluids and nutrient-rich liquids through the blood stream or directly into the stomach.

These methods can be helpful for patients who have had a stroke, ALS, MS, or esophageal cancer and need the help of a feeding tube for a period of time before going back to eating by mouth. However, a patient with a life-threatening or long-term illness may never regain the ability to eat or drink and may need the feeding tube permanently. Feeding tubes are not without risks such as pneumonia caused by regurgitated fluid in the lungs, ulcers, infections around the site, or a tube pulled out.

You may have heard withholding or withdrawal of artificial hydration and nutrition described as "starvation" or the cause of suffering before death. This is not correct. Rather, the patient's condition should be described as dehydrated. Usually, the uncomfortable symptoms of dehydration are a dry mouth and a sense of thirst. These symptoms can be alleviated with good mouth care, sips of water, or ice chips but not necessarily by artificial hydration. Medical evidence is quite clear that dehydration in the end stage of a terminal illness is a very natural and compassionate way to die.

Reasons for not using artificial hydration in a dying patient:

- Less pressure around tumors may relieve some pain.

- Less fluid in the lungs means breathing will be easier.

- Less discomfort due to fluid overload and electrolyte imbalance as the body is shutting down.

Comfort care and pain control are essential goals of any hospice team no matter what the treatment choice is regarding feeding tubes. It is important to think through and discuss these issues long before a crisis occurs. If a patient or family does not want to use a feeding tube at the end of life, it is much better not to begin the feeding at all. But if a feeding tube is started, it can be withdrawn at any time. Artificial feeding does not usually lengthen the life of a patient in the end stage of a disease; it frequently adds greater burdens. Patients can feel more isolated with artificial feeding than with hand feeding because they lose the personal interaction of someone sitting with them and feeding them.

It is understandable, however, that families struggle with decisions related to artificial feeding. They are letting go of someone important to them. From a medical viewpoint it makes sense to withhold or withdraw artificial feeding, but to a patient or family member it can be a difficult decision.

WHEN EATING AND DRINKING STOP

Eventually, favorite foods shared with family members in cheerful, homey surroundings will not interest your loved one. As your loved one's condition progresses, he will take in less food and fewer liquids. Meats are usually the first to go, followed by vegetables and other hard-to-digest foods. Eventually, eating and drinking stop.

This stage is often more upsetting for family members and friends than for the dying loved one. Dehydration is *not* painful. As the body slows down, it is less able to use nutrients and fluids. In fact, these may increase symptoms and heighten discomfort. Dying patients generally are much more comfortable without the use of artificial hydration.

These dying days can be rich with favorite people, places, and things. When feeding the body no longer brings comfort, nourish the body with your caregiving, nourish the mind with your understanding, nourish the relationship with your presence, and nourish the spirit with your love.

Financial and Legal Preparations: Getting One's House in Order

Ella and John looked over the checklist they had made to help them take care of the countless details that John's illness had brought to the forefront. As John's primary caregiver, Ella was the logical person to be given power of attorney should John no longer be able to deal with the many financial and legal decisions that had to be made. They were both so thankful for the practical guidance the hospice social worker was providing on insurance issues, financial management, wills, advance healthcare directives, and funeral arrangements. With this support they should be able to avoid any legal entanglements later on.

In addition to physical, emotional, and spiritual needs, hospice recognizes and assists with financial and legal issues as well. Limited finances, anticipated funeral expenses, and legal preparations at the end of life—all can add to a family's anxiety, hindering emotional and spiritual healing. But often the most pressing concern is the cost of caring for a terminally ill loved one at home. If you have financial or legal concerns, reach out to your hospice team. They can assist you in planning and direct you to resources that can help you pay for the care you need.

PAYING FOR HOSPICE CARE

Several programs may help pay for hospice care. These include private health insurance, Medicare, and Medicaid. Typically, hospice care at home costs less than care in a hospital. No patient will be denied hospice care because of her inability to pay. In most cases you can receive hospice care wherever you live, in a long-term care residence or assisted living facility. There may be limitations to coverage. Ask your hospice social worker.

Health Insurance

In most cases, if you have healthcare coverage through an insurance company, you are eligible for a hospice benefit. A hospice representative can contact your insurance company to ask about the specific benefits covered. It is estimated that at least eight out of ten people with employer-sponsored health plans have a hospice benefit.

Medicare

Hospice care got a big boost in 1982 when Congress made it a benefit for people who are eligible for Medicare Part A. This official recognition has made it easier for people to live their last days at home. It has provided financial and professional support, set standards to regulate professional care, and educated the helping professions as well as the public about the alternatives to dying in a hospital.

Medicare Part A covers hospital and intermittent home healthcare services and provides insurance to individuals who are sixty-five or older, disabled, or who have permanent kidney failure.

The Medicare hospice benefit, which is a separate benefit from Medicare Part A, covers hospice services. You may choose the hospice benefit if you meet all of the following criteria:

- You are eligible for Medicare Part A.

- Your physician and the hospice medical director certify in writing that you have a terminal illness with a life expectancy of six months or less if the disease runs its normal course.

- You sign an agreement with a Medicare-certified hospice (instead of accepting standard Medicare benefits for a terminal illness) and elect hospice services.

An eligible patient who is enrolled in a Medicare-managed care plan may also choose any Medicare-certified hospice provider. You can find Medicare-certified programs through your state health department, a state organization such as Hospice Minnesota, or from the National Hospice and Palliative Care Organization (NHPCO).

Services Covered under the Medicare Hospice Benefit

Hospice patients are covered under the hospice benefit for the following:

- Routine, intermittent nursing visits.

- Continuous nursing care in the home during periods of crisis as determined by the hospice team.

- Medical equipment related to the terminal illness.

- Medical supplies related to the terminal illness.

- Medications for symptom management and pain relief related to the terminal illness.

- Short-term inpatient care, including respite care.

- Home health aide and homemaker services.

- Physical, occupational, and speech therapy.

- Medical social service visits.

- Nutritional counseling and other counseling services in the home (for both patient and family).

- Spiritual care visits.

- Bereavement services for the survivors after the death of the patient.

The Medicare hospice benefit pays nearly the entire cost of these services. However, hospice may charge a small co-pay for prescriptions and for inpatient respite care.

Services NOT Covered under the Medicare Hospice Benefit

Under the hospice benefit, Medicare covers only those services authorized by the hospice program. It pays around-the-clock care only in times of medical crisis. The hospice benefit generally will not pay for:

- Aggressive treatment of a terminal illness, other than symptom management and pain control.

- Treatment of health problems unrelated to the terminal diagnosis. (These will continue to be covered under Medicare Part A or Part B.)

- Room and board at a long-term care or hospice facility.

- Additional personnel to care for your loved one for long periods of time, sometimes called "custodial care" (while you are at work, for example).

- Care provided by another hospice that was not arranged by the patient's hospice.

- Care from another provider that duplicates care the hospice is required to furnish.

- Services or treatments that have not been approved by the hospice team and are not within the hospice plan of care.

Hospice may provide other services that are not necessarily covered under the Medicare benefit. For example, programs that have music, massage, or art therapists rely on donations and memorials to provide these very valuable services.

If you are covered by both Medicare and private health insurance and you require a service that is not covered by Medicare, it might be covered by your private health insurance, and vice versa. Ask your hospice team to help you sort through your coverage options.

How Long Will Medicare Pay for Hospice?

Patients, on average, spend approximately two months in hospice care.

If you wish, you may cancel hospice care at any time, return to standard Medicare coverage, then later reelect the hospice benefit. You may also change hospice programs (if you should move, for example).

Medicare guidelines are determined by federal legislation. Because legislation changes, it is important to discuss current guidelines with your hospice team. For more information about Medicare, call 1-800-633-4227 to receive a free copy of *The Medicare Handbook.*

Medicaid

In 1986, Congress made hospice care an optional Medicaid benefit. Medicaid is a program jointly funded by the states and the federal government. It provides medical care or assistance for individuals who are unable to finance their own medical expenses. Today, more than forty states include hospice care in their Medicaid programs.

Other Reimbursement Options

Your hospice social worker will help you determine whether you are eligible for hospice benefits through Medicare or Medicaid. You might also qualify for government programs such as social security benefits, veterans' benefits, or legal aid services. Contact the Social Security Administration office, your state or local health department, or your state hospice organization for information.

Hospice programs are well known for working closely with patients and families to identify reimbursement options. Most hospices will provide services if the patient's family cannot pay, using money raised in the community or from memorials or donations.

LIFETIME PLANNING

For people receiving hospice care, the focus is no longer on fighting the disease. The goal is to focus on living—to help them live their final days comfortably, and to help them put family and business matters in order.

You and your loved one will need a notebook to record legal and financial decisions made during this time, and to write down the location of important papers and valuables. It also helps to have a folder for wills, healthcare directives, and other important documents. A document checklist can be found on page 121.

The term *lifetime planning* refers to setting up wills, joint bank accounts, powers of attorney, healthcare directives, and so forth. Your hospice social worker can provide general information about each of these. However, laws change frequently and differ from state to state, so it is best to consult an attorney or financial planner for all legal and financial matters. If affordable legal assistance is an issue, your hospice social worker can help you find out if you qualify for legal aid services.

FINANCIAL ARRANGEMENTS

Financial matters may be a source of anxiety for both you and your loved one. You can reduce this anxiety by making financial arrangements as soon as possible.

Bank Accounts

Write down all bank accounts, their locations, and their account numbers. If your loved one becomes incapacitated, it is important that a spouse, adult child, or other trusted person is able to access the person's funds to pay her bills. However, if that person shares a joint account with the loved one, it is extremely important that *only* the patient's funds enter that account. Comingled funds can create serious obstacles if the patient must later apply for Medicaid or other public assistance.

Durable Powers of Attorney

Depending on the family situation, your loved one might consider drafting a durable power of attorney. This legal document would allow a spouse, an adult child, or another trusted person to manage her financial affairs when she is no longer able. As long as your loved one is legally competent, she can revoke the power of attorney at any time. Your hospice social worker may provide a durable power of attorney form, or you can find a form on your state's Web site. Legal requirements differ from state to state, however, so it is best to consult a lawyer.

Wills and Living Trusts

With a will or living trust, your loved one can give specific instructions on how her money, property, and other assets should be distributed after she dies. She can also designate a person or persons to be responsible for distributing the estate. When people die without a will or living trust, a court must determine the distribution of their estate according to state laws. An attorney can explain the laws in your state.

Wills must include the name of a personal representative (executor of the will) and instructions for distributing the patient's property. A will should be signed and witnessed by two people in the presence of the author (testator) and each other. Each witness should also include his or her address. The author should sign all pages of the will and not make any changes after it has been witnessed. Requirements for legal wills vary from state to state, so ask about the specific requirements in your state.

A holographic will is a will that is handwritten by the author, signed, and dated. No witnesses are required. Such wills are legal in several states. Your social worker can tell you if they are legal in your state.

Probate is a legal process that transfers property from a deceased person's estate to her beneficiaries. Generally, probate can be completed in one year. Even with a will, it is likely that some of the estate will go through probate.

A living trust allows property to pass to beneficiaries without going through probate. Unlike a will, this process is fast and private. It is important to note, however, that a living trust may affect eligibility for Medicaid benefits. Talk to an attorney before creating a living trust.

Intestate is a term describing a person who dies without a will or living trust. If a loved one dies intestate, her property will usually go first to the surviving spouse, then to the loved one's children, and then to other blood relatives. Without a will or living trust, long delays may occur in settling the estate, and the government may end up with a much larger part of it.

Write down the location of the original will, living trust, or estate plan. You should also give copies of the document to one or two other family members or trusted friends. Attach a note indicating where the original copy can be found.

If your loved one's estate is large, talk to an attorney or financial planner about how to limit federal and state taxes. If your loved one's finances are depleted, a will is still a good idea. She can specify how family treasures—photo albums, jewelry, or favorite antiques, for example—should be divided. This may prevent quarrels among family members after her death.

Other Financial Matters

Your loved one should write down information about her stocks and bonds, social security or veterans' benefits, pensions, and insurance policies (noting location, kind of policy, amount, settlement options available, and status of any loans against the policies). If your loved one has a safe-deposit box, it is important to note the location of the box and key, as well as the contents of the box.

AARP (formerly, the American Association of Retired Persons) suggests other steps you and your loved one can take to protect her assets and avoid legal entanglements:

- Make sure all joint assets accurately reflect who owns what. Have all appropriate names recorded.

- To change the name on a deed, contact the registrar of deeds in the county where the property is located.

- Remove the dying person's name from jointly held stocks or bonds. Add the names of other appropriate people, such as children.

- Remove the dying person's name from joint bank accounts. Inform the bank of what is happening.

- If survivors are covered under your loved one's health insurance, check to see how long they will be covered after the patient's death. If necessary, obtain health insurance for the survivors.

- Transfer the title of the dying person's automobile and home.

- Ask the dying person where any other assets might be located.

If assets are transferred *after* your loved one dies, taxes may be higher, and survivors may have to wait until the will and estate go through probate. It is best to take care of these matters while your loved one is still alive. However, it is usually wise to consult with an estate attorney in order to understand all the ramifications.

HEALTHCARE DECISIONS

A duly executed will and a law can permit physicians, hospitals and nursing homes to honor a person's desires without legal repercussions.

—Jane E. Brody, "Personal Health"

Although hospice focuses on comfort care instead of a cure, life-threatening medical conditions may arise, such as pneumonia. The question then becomes whether to treat the condition. It is best to discuss this issue *before* such a condition arises, while your loved one is still able to make decisions.

Competent adults have the right to make their own healthcare decisions, including whether to accept, reject, or discontinue specific kinds of medical care. However, there may come a time when your loved one cannot express her wishes. This is why it's a good idea to have a living will, advance healthcare directive, or durable power of attorney for healthcare.

Durable Powers of Attorney for Healthcare

A durable power of attorney for healthcare names a trusted family member or friend to make medical decisions on the patient's behalf if she becomes incapacitated. The patient can list specific instructions in the document. These instructions should address the same issues as a living will or advance healthcare directive. Talk to your hospice social worker about your state's rules regarding durable powers of attorney for healthcare.

Living Wills and Advance Healthcare Directives

A living will is a legal document stating an individual's wishes regarding life-sustaining treatment if she goes into a vegetative state with no hope of recovery. A recent poll showed that 90 percent of people, when presented with this scenario, would not want to be kept alive on an artificial life-support system, yet fewer than 25 percent have a living will.

Living wills are legal in at least forty states. Talk to your hospice social worker to see if they are legal in your state. Send a copy of your loved one's living will to her primary doctor, attorney, and hospice agency. Also, keep a copy in the patient's home as health care providers may request a copy.

An advance healthcare directive is a formal document, written by a competent person, to guide medical treatment if that person becomes mentally incapacitated. The 1991 Patient Self-Determination Act requires all U.S. hospitals, nursing facilities, health maintenance organizations (HMOs), and other healthcare delivery systems to ask incoming patients if they have an advance healthcare directive (or living will) or whether they wish to complete one. In addition, healthcare agencies, including hospices, that receive federal funds are required to inform all patients of their right to refuse or consent to treatment. Unfortunately, by the time some people are admitted to a hospital, they may not be competent and able to make their wishes known.

What to Consider in an Advance Healthcare Directive

Most living wills or advance healthcare directives address

- Intravenous or tube feeding (nutrition),

- Intravenous fluids (hydration),

- Cardiopulmonary resuscitation (CPR),

- Mechanical ventilation,

- Antibiotics,

- Blood transfusions,

- Kidney dialysis,

- Donation of body.

An attorney can help you tailor your living will to fit your specific needs.

The Benefits of Living Wills and Advance Healthcare Directives

Janis, a sixty-six-year-old grandmother, prepared a living will after she was diagnosed with cancer. Three months later she was hospitalized with kidney failure. As she specified in her living will, Janis did not want dialysis. She wanted to die as peacefully and comfortably as possible, so a "Do Not Resuscitate" (DNR) notice was placed on her chart. Hours later, after saying goodbye to relatives and friends, she slipped quietly into a coma. Her heart and breathing stopped shortly after that.

Janis wanted to spare her family the terror she felt ten years ago when her sister died of cancer. During her sister's last hours, she watched as tubes and machines sustained a shell of a person toward no meaningful end.

While documents such as advance healthcare directives or living wills are very important, it is equally important for patients to discuss their wishes with their family, friends, and other loved ones. In addition to consulting directives, healthcare providers will always look to family for guidance when patients are unable to speak for themselves.

PLANNING THE FUNERAL OR MEMORIAL

One of the most meaningful ways to take control of the dying process is to plan the funeral or memorial service. Although such an open acknowledgment of death may be difficult, there are a great many advantages to making arrangements beforehand. For one thing, it assures a remembrance unique to your loved one. The hospice spiritual care provider can be of great assistance in this area.

With funeral or memorial plans in place, the family and the loved one can concentrate on the social and spiritual aspects of grieving and remembering. Planning ahead also frees the family from having to make weighty decisions at a difficult time. Even if death has been anticipated, many families are surprised by the intensity of their grief.

Funeral or memorial plans can be a difficult topic to bring up. Your hospice nurse, social worker, or spiritual care provider can help open discussions between your loved one and family members. They can also put you in touch with funeral directors in the area.

Funeral directors are becoming more sensitive toward clients' desire to control the funeral process. Many funeral directors will visit patients and their families at home or in the hospital. And a federal regulation called the Funeral Rule helps ensure that families know which funeral and burial options are available and how much they will cost. The rule requires funeral homes (but not cemeteries) to give prices by telephone and offer price lists for review.

Before making any decisions, get itemized, written estimates. Every funeral home should have separate price lists for general services, caskets, and outer burial containers. Use all three lists to determine the total cost of the funeral. Don't be shamed into spending more than you can afford. Price is not a measure of your feelings for your loved one.

Although making funeral plans at some point prior to death may be less stressful, do not worry if you don't have plans in place when death occurs. Even when someone is terminally ill, death can be somewhat unexpected. You can make funeral arrangements at any time. However, at some point before death, your hospice nurse will need to know the name of the mortuary.

Burial or Cremation

Your loved one should decide whether she wishes to be buried or cremated. Once you've made the decision, add this information to your advance healthcare directive. If in-ground burial is the choice, you and your loved one must select a cemetery plot.

Cremation is becoming an increasingly popular choice. It is simple, and cost effective. The ashes might be buried, placed in a cemetery niche, scattered over some special place, or kept in a family member's home.

Visitation

In many American traditions, a visitation is often held the evening before (or an hour or two before) a traditional funeral. It is an opportunity for friends and relatives to pay their respects and lend support to the family. Whether to have an open casket is another decision you and your loved one must make. If the casket will be open, you might discuss what your loved one would like to be wearing. Some families choose not to have a visitation.

Funeral or Memorial Service

The traditional funeral takes place in a church, synagogue, temple, or mortuary. Again, whether to have an open casket depends on your loved one's preference. Some people prefer a closed casket so others will remember them as they were when alive. Others prefer an open casket to help loved ones confront the reality of death. A traditional funeral will require you and your loved one to choose six to eight pallbearers. They can be relatives or friends.

A memorial service is similar to a funeral except the casket is not present. If your loved one was cremated, you may choose to have the urn present. Whether you plan a traditional funeral or a memorial service, several decisions should be made ahead of time:

- Who will be notified of the death (relatives, friends, business associates)?

- Who can make the calls?

- What kind of printed memorial will be given to those attending the visitation/funeral/memorial?

- Will there be a guest book? If so, who will be in charge?

- How can you best celebrate the life of the loved one?

- Who will preside over the service?

- What music is to be played or sung?

- Who is to speak?

- If there are children, how can they be involved? Might they draw pictures to be placed in the casket?

- Will there be a graveside service? Public or private?

- Will there be a reception following the service? If so, where?

- Will refreshments be served?

- Will photographs of the loved one be displayed?

- What will be done with the flowers after the service?

The Obituary

Many people with terminal illnesses appreciate the opportunity to write their own obituary (death notice). They might include statements about their life, work, and interests. An obituary should list the names of the loved one, deceased family members, and survivors.

It should also note whether memorials are preferred instead of flowers. Some families request donations to a favorite charity, organization, or place of worship. Many others direct memorials to their hospice. Hospices rely on memorials to help families who cannot afford necessary services. The memorials may also be used for staff and volunteer education and bereavement matters, as well as special services not covered by insurance.

When death occurs, the details regarding the person's age, time of death, and funeral or memorial arrangements can be added to the obituary. Decide which newspapers and other publications should receive the information.

Paying for the Funeral, Memorial, and/or Burial

Funerals, memorial services, and burials can be paid for in advance (through a trust or payment plan), or after death (by life insurance). A member of the hospice team, typically the social worker, can put you in touch with someone to advise you of your options. Find out if a deposit or prepayment has been made on any part of the funeral or burial. If a cemetery plot exists, have the title or deed to this plot in your "Important Documents" folder.

OTHER FINAL PREPARATIONS

Some people with terminal illnesses list all their unfinished projects and put them into priority order. Whether they complete their projects alone or ask a family member or friend to help, they begin to approach a sense of closure. For example, some people write poems or letters to their loved ones. Others make audio- or videotapes to share their thoughts and love with those they will leave behind.

Your loved one may wish to investigate the possibility of donating organs—or even her body—to medical science. This, too, can bring a sense of accomplishment through death. The hospice team can give you information to help with this decision.

Your loved one may wish to have a religious ceremony, such as the Anointing of the Sick (last rites), performed before she dies. Discuss the details of your loved one's wishes, then contact your hospice spiritual care provider or a leader in your faith community. He or she can help you make the proper arrangements.

If your loved one is a single parent with dependent children, the issue of guardianship must be addressed. The hospice team or an attorney can help your loved one express her wishes legally in order to prevent family quarrels and other difficulties. In addition, your loved one might want to write letters to her children. These letters might be opened when the children reach a certain age and can better understand death and dying.

You must also find out who has the authority to pronounce your loved one dead and to sign the death certificate. Some states allow a hospice nurse to do this, while other states require a physician or a coroner.

Tying up as many loose ends as possible fills the days with meaningful activity and is an important step toward letting go of life peacefully.

DOCUMENT CHECKLIST

_____ address book
_____ advance healthcaredirective
_____ automobile titles or leases
_____ bank statements (checking, savings, line of credit)
_____ birth certificate
_____ bonds
_____ burial plot or cemetery information
_____ credit/debit cards
_____ deeds to property
_____ document authorizing donation of body
_____ driver's license
_____ employment history
_____ funeral/cremation arrangements, prepayments
_____ health insurance policies
_____ income tax returns
_____ inventory of possessions
_____ life insurance policies
_____ living trust
_____ living will
_____ loans
_____ marriage certificate
_____ Medicare ID card
_____ membership lists
_____ military discharge papers
_____ mortgage papers (including any mortgage insurance)
_____ organ donor card
_____ pension or retirement plans
_____ powers of attorney (general, durable healthcare)
_____ property and casualty insurance
_____ safety deposit box (list of contents and location of keys)
_____ savings bonds
_____ Social Security card
_____ stock certificates
_____ valuables (complete inventory and locations of items)
_____ Veterans' Administration papers
_____ will

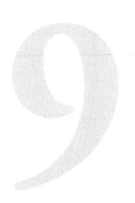

When Death Is Near:
Your Final Days Together

> *When someone dies, it is important that those close*
> *to him participate in the process; it will help them in*
> *their grief, and it will help them face their own*
> *death more easily.*
>
> —Elisabeth Kübler-Ross

Ella squeezed John's hand as he labored to breathe. They both knew time was short. Family members had already gathered together and said their goodbyes. John whispered, "I love you, Ella," and she responded, "I love you too." He closed his eyes and drifted off to sleep. Soon after, his breathing stopped, and Ella knew he had died. She called the family in and asked son Tim to call the hospice nurse and let her know that John had died. Then, family members took turns saying their private goodbyes, each in his or her own way.

Completing the circle of life can be very difficult. Helping your loved one finish this journey may be the hardest, and perhaps the most rewarding, challenge you will ever face. Your caregiving, support, and love will be of utmost importance as your loved one begins a journey that only he can truly experience and understand. In hospice, it is possible to accompany your loved one to the very end of his or her journey through life. Hospice also offers a unique chance to surround your loved one with tangible proof of his value to others and to focus on what the present day has to offer.

ALTERNATIVE CARE OPTIONS

In some instances, care at home becomes too difficult, and families must find alternate care for their loved one. In other cases, patients are already living in a long-term care residence when they are diagnosed with a terminal illness. The majority of people in the United States die in a hospital or other care facility.

Patients can receive hospice care wherever they live, whether in their home, an inpatient hospice residence, a nursing home, a long-term care residence, or assisted living facility. Remember, hospice is not a place of service—it is a philosophy of care. In fact, many hospices have contracts with long-term care facilities to provide hospice care.

If you move your loved one to long-term care, your hospice social worker will assist you. Although the staff will become the primary caregivers, you can continue to provide love and support, and your hospice team will continue to manage your loved one's hospice care.

If your loved one already lives in a long-term care facility and is not yet enrolled in a hospice program, ask the facility's social worker to help you choose a hospice.

Together, the hospice and long-term care facility will establish a coordinated care plan. The hospice will educate the staff about hospice philosophy and procedures, and about caring for the terminally ill. The facility will provide room and board, offer social activities, administer medications, and assist with personal care. The hospice and facility staff will collaborate closely to ensure that your loved one's needs are being met. The hospice will be notified if there is a change in your loved one's condition, and the facility will be notified if there is a change in the hospice care plan.

If your loved one is covered under the Medicare hospice benefit, this benefit will not cover custodial care or room and board in a facility. These services will have to be paid for. If your family has no applicable insurance or cannot afford to pay for these services, the hospice team will help you apply for Medicaid or other financial assistance.

If your loved one will receive hospice care in a long-term care facility, it is extremely important to make his advanced directives known, especially regarding nutrition, hydration, hospitalization, and specific medical conditions. For example, you and your loved one should decide what to do if he comes down with pneumonia. Pneumonia has been called "the friend of the dying" and is often viewed as a blessing. It is seldom painful and causes the body to shut down before more difficult symptoms can cause death. On the other hand, pneumonia could cut short days or weeks that are precious to you both.

If it is important for your loved one to remain at home, ask the hospice nurse or social worker about the option of hiring home health aides or nurses to come to your home to help with caregiving. This is commonly called "custodial care."

INVOLVING CHILDREN

Children can be deeply affected by the illness and death of a loved one. Depending on their ages, children may or may not be able to express their feelings. Following are some suggestions for helping children cope with death:

- Be open about what's happening. Children can tell if you are keeping something from them, and your secrecy may make them think they're responsible for their loved one's illness or death.

- Listen to children, preferably at their eye level, and answer questions honestly and briefly. It's okay to say that you don't know all the answers.

- Help children say goodbye to their loved one. If you're not sure whether they should go to the funeral, share your concerns and allow them to make the final decision.

- Ask the child to tell you what is happening. This will tell you if the child has a clear understanding of the events that are taking place.

- Avoid clichés such as "Grandma went to sleep" or "God needs Daddy more than we do." Use the terms *death* and *dying*.

- Remind children of happy memories. Tell them it's okay to remember their loved one and to say his name.

- Ask your hospice team or religious community about support groups and other resources to help children and parents through the grieving process.

WHEN YOUR LOVED ONE WANTS TO HASTEN DEATH

As the end draws near, your loved one may want to hasten his death. One of the most common reasons for wanting to die quickly is uncontrolled pain. Your hospice team can help with uncontrolled pain. If pain is the reason for talk of suicide or euthanasia (assisted, painless death), communicate this urgent concern to your hospice nurse so progressive pain-control measures can be put in place.

Another reason your loved one might want to die sooner is because he feels like a burden. It is important to reassure your loved one. Explain that you want to have as many days together as possible, and that you truly enjoy being able to care for his needs.

Loss of dignity and control is another reason your loved one may talk of suicide or euthanasia. Incontinence (loss of bladder or bowel control), for example, can be humiliating and embarrassing for anyone. If it has been going on for several days or weeks, your loved one may want it to end—now. Again, assure your loved one that you understand. If your loved one does not have a urinary catheter, this might be a good time to talk with the hospice nurse about this option. Let your loved one make as many decisions as possible so he feels more in control of other areas in his life. Talk to your hospice social worker or spiritual care provider about other ways to comfort and reassure your loved one.

No matter what the underlying issues, if your loved one wants to hasten death, you need not be shocked, and you need not consent. Discuss the alternatives. Talk about how precious each day can be and all the things you can still share together.

REMAINING CLOSE UNTIL THE END

It is often difficult to be with a person who is approaching death. You may want to plan for more support during these final days. Usually, the hospice nurse and other team members will visit more often in the days just before death.

Caregivers are often action-oriented, juggling numerous responsibilities at any given time. As a caregiver, you may find it difficult to just sit and talk with your loved one. At this point, however, your presence is the most important thing you can give. Be a good listener. Acknowledge that you understand your loved one's concerns. Use the positive approach. Repeat what you have heard in a tone of voice that shows acceptance. "I understand that you are angry. Do you want to talk about it?" Listen and accept what your loved one is saying as his truth. If you are having difficulties with these conversations, talk with the hospice social worker about your concerns.

Ask, "How are you feeling—really?" And wait for the honest answer. Don't be uncomfortable with long periods of silence. Silence can be golden. It may be tiring for your loved one to talk or even to listen.

It's okay to talk about dying and the symptoms you are probably both noticing. If your loved one asks questions you can't answer, admit that you don't know, then ask your hospice team for the information. If your loved one asks, "Why me?" tell the truth: probably, "I don't know." If your loved one asks point blank, "Am I dying now?" say what is in your heart. You might ask, "Do you think you are?" or "Does it feel like you are?" Reassure your loved one that he is alive now and that's what's important.

Try to maintain a sense of humor, and don't argue over trivial things. Assure your loved one that he is not alone. Keep your loved one clean, dry, and warm. Now is a time to touch, hug, and kiss.

Your loved one will resent being treated like a child. He probably doesn't want to be "taken care of" any more than is absolutely necessary. Let your loved one be the "boss." Ask what he would like to do or to have done so that he can remain in control as much as possible.

Be gentle, slow, reliable, honest, and permissive. Do not over-schedule your loved one. Be flexible. The most important schedule now is the pain medication schedule.

During these final days you will probably want fewer visitors and fewer distractions. Gentle background music can mask the extraneous sounds and set a serene mood. If you have a music therapist, ask for suggestions on music selections. Silence might also be good at this time. When visitors or family members come, do not whisper, and do not talk behind your loved one's back. Also, ask them not to speak in front of your loved one as if he isn't there. Even if your loved one appears to be asleep, he may hear the conversation and feel distressed at being left out. If your loved one is in a coma, he may still hear you. Talk as you would if your loved one was conscious, especially if there are unfinished things to say. Say them and believe that they are heard.

Try to arrange for someone to be with your loved one—although sometimes a dying person may need to be alone. Do not stop the pain medications. If your loved one becomes unable to swallow, talk to your hospice nurse about alternate forms of pain control, such as sublingual (under the tongue) or by patch. Do *not* force foods or liquids. This may cause discomfort because the body is shutting down and cannot process them.

You may find yourself feeling angry that death is taking so long. This anger is normal. Forgive yourself for having these feelings. You may feel bad if you are not there at the precise moment of death. Again, forgive yourself. This may be your loved one's expression of love for you. Some caregivers suggest that their loved one's final gift was to die when they were not present, sparing them from the pain and sorrow likely to be felt at the moment of death.

One hospice volunteer went every Wednesday to be with a dying man so the man's wife and daughter could go shopping. The volunteer knew the man didn't want to talk, but he went anyway, knowing how important the respite was for the caregivers. This went on for several weeks. One Wednesday, when the volunteer went to check on the man shortly after the wife and daughter had left, he found that the man had died. The volunteer was able to call together the hospice team and the rest of the family and have them waiting there when the wife and daughter returned.

Death Anxiety

When death is near, you and your loved one may become frightened. This is normal. Most people are not afraid of being dead; they are afraid of the moment of death. Read about the signs of approaching death so you know what to look for.

Letting Go

During the last few days, your attitude needs to be one of letting go, of releasing your loved one, of letting your loved one know that you'll be okay. All you can do now is be there and reassure your loved one that he will be deeply missed but not forgotten. Your loved one may try to hang on, wanting to be persuaded that those left behind will be all right. Give your permission to let go. Your ability to reassure and release your loved one is the greatest love you can show. This is what you would want from your loved one if your roles were reversed.

Saying Goodbye

Each person will have his or her own way of saying goodbye. It's okay to lie in bed with your loved one, holding his hand and saying everything you need to say. Tears are natural at this time. Let them flow. Don't try to hide them or apologize for them. They are an expression of your love. If you are not present when your loved one dies, be kind and forgiving to yourself. Your loved one may have wanted to be alone or wanted to protect you. Do not blame yourself or your loved one.

SIGNS OF APPROACHING DEATH

The transition from life can be every bit as pro-
found, intimate and precious as the miracle of birth.

—Ira R. Byock

During the terminal phase, the body experiences an orderly, undramatic series of physical changes as it begins the final process of shutting down. On the emotional-spiritual plane, the spirit of the dying person begins the final process of release from the body, its environment, and all its attachments. If your loved one has unresolved conflicts, unkept promises, unfinished projects, or damaged relationships, he may have trouble letting go. Help your loved one come to grips with any unfinished business.

The following discussion provides a general idea of what you might expect. It is not meant to alarm you, but to prepare you for what might happen. As death approaches, your loved one may experience some or all of the signs. Active dying may take hours or days; the signs may appear and disappear. Active dying can be physically and emotionally draining for you and your loved one. It is important to understand that these signs of impending death are normal. Do not be alarmed by them, and don't allow them to alarm your loved one.

Mental and Emotional Signs

As your loved one prepares to die, he may begin to withdraw. Your loved one may start shutting out television, newspapers, magazines, friends, family members, and even you. This is a sign that your loved one is beginning to focus inward. Even when he appears to be asleep, important work is going on inside. Withdrawal can be difficult for family members, but it is normal. It is a time of silent reflection on the meaning of life and impending death.

Don't interpret withdrawal as lack of love; your loved one is simply starting the dying process. Your presence is still important. If your loved one wants to be alone most of the time or with only one person, respect his wishes, but continue to make your care and love known.

At this point, many caregiving tasks may no longer be necessary or appropriate. Keep your loved one comfortable, perhaps moistening his lips with cool water, holding his hand, and offering reassurance: "I'm here for you. I'll be with you."

Extreme anxiety or restlessness is another sign of impending death. Your loved one may pick at bedclothes or linens. He may make repetitive motions, pulling at clothes or sheets. Do not restrain these actions. Talk calmly and quietly about whatever comes to mind. Try to distract your loved one with something he enjoys, such as music or television. You might talk with the hospice nurse about medications to relieve his anxiety and restlessness.

Your loved one may become confused about what day it is, what time it is, or who people are. Disorientation is usually a result of changes in metabolism. Gently reorient your loved one each morning by stating what day and time it is. Announce yourself when you enter the room. When family members or friends visit, announce their names as well. Explain what you are doing each time you assist your loved one, for example, "It's time to take your pills now so you won't have any pain."

Your loved one may hallucinate. He may talk to God or to people you do not see. In several instances, dying people have been reported to see and converse with others who have died before them. Your loved one may talk of "going home," referring to an afterlife. Behavior like this may be a result of decreased oxygen to the brain. Do not interfere with your loved one. Listen to what he is saying. You may learn something important.

Physical Signs

As death approaches, the body loses the ability to maintain itself. Your loved one may grow weak and move around less. He may experience a gradual loss of sensation. As the circulation slows, skin may be cool to the touch, especially on the arms and legs. It may feel clammy, and the underside of the body may become darker. The skin may turn a bluish, mottled color. Fingernails and toenails may become pale and blue.

Your loved one's temperature may fluctuate between hot and cold, accompanied by changes in skin color: flushed with fever and bluish with cold. Perspiration may increase. Adjust your loved one's blankets as the body temperature changes. Do not use an electric blanket.

You may notice some involuntary jerking or twitching in the arms, legs, or facial muscles. This may be the result of decreased circulation, a buildup of waste products in the body, or high doses of pain medications. These motions are not painful or uncomfortable.

Breathing patterns may change. While 16 to 20 breaths per minute is considered normal, your loved one may take as many as 40 or 50 breaths per minute, or as few as 6. Breathing may stop entirely for a few moments and then begin again. Your hospice physician and nurse may refer to this as apnea. This symptom is very common and results from a decrease in circulation and a buildup of body wastes. Elevating the head of the bed might make breathing easier. If your loved one has trouble breathing, you may want to ask your hospice nurse about oxygen. Sometimes a tranquilizer can help. Lip balm or a dab of petroleum jelly might alleviate dryness caused by breathing through the mouth. Ice chips, water through a straw, and cool moist washcloths may relieve the feelin of dehydration.

Oral secretions may increase and collect at the back of the throat, causing a gurgling sound when your loved one breathes. This symptom results from a decrease in fluids and an inability to cough up normal saliva and mucous. It is sometimes called the "death rattle." Although the sound may be distressing to you and others, your loved one may not even notice it. Elevating the head may ease this symptom. You might also talk with your hospice nurse about oxygen or medication for this type of breathing.

Blood pressure may drop. The pulse rate may rise from a normal 80 beats per minute to 150 beats per minute, or it may drop to almost zero.

Vision and hearing may decrease slightly. Keep the lights on if vision has decreased, and never assume that your loved one cannot hear you. Hearing is usually the last of the five senses to go. Get close to your loved one when you are talking so he can hear you.

Your loved one may eat and drink even less than before, perhaps stopping entirely. This is okay. You might offer small amounts of food or fluids, but do not insist. The output of urine may decrease and darken. This concentrated urine is caused by decreased fluid intake and decreased circulation through the kidneys. Another sign of approaching death is incontinence—losing control of the bladder and/or bowels. If this occurs, use disposable pads and diapers. The hospice nurse can show you some techniques to aid hygiene.

Talk with the nurse about catheter placement. If your loved one already has a catheter, inform your hospice nurse as urine output decreases—the catheter may need to be irrigated to prevent blockage.

Changes in the body's metabolism may cause your loved one to spend more and more time sleeping, and you might find it difficult to wake him up. Or, your loved one may drift into semiconsciousness and sleep almost constantly for days before he dies. It is also possible that your loved one will be conscious and talking until moments before death.

WHEN DEATH IS VERY NEAR

When your loved one is close to death, these symptoms may intensify. Breathing patterns may become even more irregular. Congestion may become more pronounced. Restlessness could increase markedly. A yellow pallor might appear. Your loved one's eyes may stare, open but unseeing. They might look glassy or teary. The pupils may react less to light. The hands and feet may become purplish, and the ankles, knees, and elbows might look blotchy. If it has not already happened, urinary or bowel incontinence may occur. You might notice brown secretions in the mouth—old blood, possibly from the stomach lining. The body may have an odor. And you may have great difficulty awakening your loved one.

When you feel death is very near, you might want to call the family together. They may have things they want to say to your loved one. You should also inform your hospice team members.

Near death, your loved one may have a burst of energy; he might even want to talk or eat. This may appear to be a spiritual energy that has arrived to help your loved one transition from life to death.

Your loved one may or may not be conscious right up to the moment of death. Often, people slip into death just as easily as they fall asleep each night. If your loved one becomes very restless, medications can help with this symptom.

THE MOMENT OF DEATH

A moment—that's how long it takes for your loved one to leave his physical body. Death usually occurs when the body finishes shutting down and your loved one has reconciled important issues or resolved relationship problems. You'll know that your loved one has died when he stops breathing for several minutes and the heart is no longer beating. If the eyelids are open, the eyes will remain in a fixed stare. The mouth may fall open. The bowels and bladder may empty.

This is not the time to panic and call 9-1-1. The emergency response team would only attempt to resuscitate your loved one because that is what they are trained to do. Remember your loved one's wishes regarding resuscitation, and let your loved one go. If someone unexpectedly calls 9-1-1 and you have a signed DNR (Do Not Resuscitate) form, have it available and ready for the paramedics. Keep this form accessible at all times.

IMMEDIATELY AFTER DEATH

Note the time of death and call your hospice nurse. He or she will contact the appropriate authorities. The nurse can also remove the catheter, if one is present, and help you dispose of medications. The hospice nurse will know who is authorized to pronounce your loved one dead and sign the death certificate.

If your loved one had made a decision to donate his body or specific organs for research, ask the hospice nurse for further instructions.

If the eyes are open, you might gently close the lids. If the mouth has dropped open, you might prop the head up with a pillow so the mouth closes. If dentures were removed, you might want to put them back in before the jaw becomes rigid.

The body will gradually cool, turn pale, and stiffen over several hours. You may wish to bathe and dress the body before it stiffens. It's okay to touch and caress the body, but understand that your loved one is no longer there. Spend enough time with the body to know that it's only an empty shell now. Do whatever feels right. Pray. Cry. Hold someone. Have someone hold you. Then, call your relatives and friends and set your funeral, memorial, and/or burial plans into motion.

Many families prefer to keep the body in the home for a few hours. Some people have an informal wake, gathering family and friends to say goodbye and to reminisce about their loved one's life.

THE END OF A JOURNEY

Death is the conclusion of the journey you have made with your loved one to his final rest. It will be sad. It will hurt. But it should also be comforting to know that you and your loved one have successfully completed the journey together.

> *I am standing upon the seashore. A ship at my side spreads her white sails to the morning breeze and starts for the blue ocean. She is an object of beauty and strength. I stand and watch her until at length she hangs like a speck of white cloud just where the sea and sky come to mingle with each other.*
>
> *Then someone at my side says: "There, she is gone!"*
>
> *"Gone where?"*
>
> *Gone from my sight. That is all.*
>
> *Her diminished size is in me, not in her. And just at the moment when someone at my side says: "There, she is gone!" there are other eyes watching her coming, and other voices ready to take up the glad shout: "Here she comes!"*
>
> *And that is dying.*
>
> —Henry Van Dyke

10

After the Loss: Moving On

Death is not extinguishing the light; it is putting out
the lamp because dawn has come.

—Tagore

Ella sat quietly on the first anniversary of John's death listening to their
favorite song. She and John had shared that special song throughout
their married lives. It had taken months before she could bear to play
it. Now it was comforting. Her life would never be the same. How
could it be when such a large part of it was taken from her? But she
had so much to be grateful for: their years together, their children, her
health, her friends—old and new—and the help of hospice during a
very difficult year. The doorbell rang and there stood her son Tim and
his family. They had come to take her to dinner on this significant day.

The death of a loved one can be devastating. Knowing that
death is inevitable—and maybe even desired—does not diminish
the grief you feel. In fact, you probably started grieving while your
loved one was still alive.

At first there are many details to take care of, both personal and
financial. Family and friends visit often and include you in their
get-togethers. In time, however, they return to their normal routine
and you are left to deal with your grief. But you are not alone.
Hospice bereavement services will help you through your grief and
provide you with a list of support options.

This chapter not only addresses the practical matters that must be attended to, but also explains the grieving process to help you work through your pain and grief.

GRIEF

> Grief is like a wound. At first, it's open, bleeding, raw and terribly painful. In time that wound begins to heal. It heals from the inside out. The pain begins to fade and eventually a scar is formed . . . . There will always be a scar. We will never be the same again.
>
> —Barbara Karnes, "My Friend, I Care"

Grief is a reaction to loss. You grieve not only for your loved one, but also for yourself and your disrupted world. You may grieve over lost companionship, lost opportunities, and lost dreams.

To further complicate matters, you may find yourself alternating between feelings of grief for your loss and relief that the struggle is over. Although grieving may seem irrational at times, you are not going crazy.

All the "firsts" will be difficult—the first birthday, Thanksgiving, wedding anniversary, and death anniversary. For a while, your grief will seem all-consuming. You will imagine your loved one's reaction to every event; you will want to share every piece of news, good or bad.

You may be afraid of the future, of life without your loved one. But you won't be without your loved one. You will always have your memories and feel that special love you shared. Only the body is gone.

You may fear that you will also die, perhaps leaving your children alone. You may fear that others you love will die. All of this is normal. Death makes us realize how fragile life is.

The Grieving Process

The loss of a loved one affects many aspects of a person's life. For example, if we lose a spouse, we may also lose a lover, a travel companion, a coparent, and a best friend.

—Steve Sims, hospice bereavement coordinator

Grieving is a unique, personal process. There are still people who expect grieving to last one year. This is not always realistic. In a society such as ours, encompassing many cultural traditions, there is no norm. Some people grieve for a shorter time, others for longer, and some forever. The following discussion of the grieving process is only a guide. You may not experience each aspect of grief in the order described. Just as with Kübler-Ross's stages of dying, you may skip a stage, or you might get stuck in a stage. You might go through every stage and then regress. The description herein will simply help you understand the various aspects of grief you might experience after the death of your loved one.

The first phase of grief is usually one of shock and denial. You may feel dazed, numb, bewildered, angry, and hostile. You may react with disbelief even though you knew it was coming. You might go on autopilot, taking care of arrangements and keeping very busy. Your heart may race, your stomach may ache, you might become dizzy and light-headed. This stage is a sort of buffer from the reality that you will eventually face. It will wear off.

Another phase is one of searching for connections to your loved one. You may sense her presence and expect to hear a call for your help. You might talk to your loved one; you might even think that you hear or see your loved one. This, too, is normal.

Despair and disorientation characterize yet another stage in the grieving process. As reality sets in, you may feel helpless, uncertain, and fearful. You may feel angry and look for someone to blame for your loss. You don't want to change. You don't want to be alone. You might feel guilty, blaming yourself for not having done everything possible for your loved one. You may question your faith. You might be confused, depressed, and withdrawn. You might feel a loss of identity or self-worth. You may find yourself wandering aimlessly around the house or starting projects and forgetting to finish them. You may need to tell the story of your loved one and her death over and over again. Your mood may change with the slightest provocation and you may cry uncontrollably at unexpected times.

The final phase of grief is one of adapting, recovering, reorienting, and accepting. Like death, grief is a natural part of life. You may wake up feeling relatively happy; then a salesperson will call and ask for your loved one, and your whole world will come crashing down again. Getting to the acceptance stage—and staying there—is a long, slow process.

The Physical Impact of Grief

Grief can take a toll on you physically. You may lose interest or gain interest in food. You may lose weight. You may have intense dreams or disturbing sleep patterns—if you can sleep at all. You may be extremely restless, unable to concentrate or relax. Furthermore, grief can hurt: You might feel a knot in your stomach, a tightness in your throat, or a heaviness in your chest. Often grief requires more energy than you would need to chop wood. You may require lots of rest to maintain your health.

The Emotional Toll of Grief

As your loved one is dying, you may feel grief, anger, denial, isolation, depression, and many other emotions. When death comes, you may feel relief. The house is quiet. Your job is done. But this sense of relief might indicate that you are numb and in a state of shock—the first stage of grief. Grief is a powerful, painful emotion. Loneliness may be a constant companion for a long time, even when other people are around. If your loved one was your spouse, you may feel an emptiness, a huge void that some people refer to as the "dark night of the soul." This void, however, serves a purpose: As the ancient Zen saying points out, "You can't fill a teacup that's already full." Accept the emptiness, knowing that you can grow a new life there when the time is right. Do not try to fill the emptiness with meaningless activity. Use it to work through your loss. You may want to request help with this from your hospice bereavement counselor.

Some people experience little or no distress or grief after a loved one dies. In fact, one researcher found that it is common for grief to be "borne lightly." This can be a sign of resilience, of a deep, enduring love. Belief in a higher power may also lessen grief, allowing you to see death as part of life's grand plan. If you do not feel distress or grief, others may think you are cold or unloving. More likely, they will think you are hiding your true feelings, toughing it out. But it doesn't matter what others think.

Expressing Grief

> *A person's grief is as unique as their fingerprint.*
> *No two people grieve in the same way or at the*
> *same time.*
>
> —Steve Sims, hospice bereavement coordinator

It doesn't matter how you express your grief, only that you do. Cry, yell, scream, stomp around, sob softly, sit in silence. Cry as much as you want to—it's a good release for those pent-up feelings. Do whatever feels right. Don't try to be strong if you don't feel like it. Handle your grief in your own way. You may want to be very open about your grief, or you may try to hide it. You may try to avoid your grief by keeping busy. You may hold your grief back, fearing that once you start grieving you won't be able to stop. Friends may give you advice—keep a stiff upper lip, get on with your life, and so forth. They mean well, but only you know how best to grieve your loss.

Recognize, however, that grief may become excessive—too intense or too prolonged. Although grief is necessary, it can become a trap, a habit of suffering. Don't get stuck in grief. Seek counseling, join a support group, talk to the hospice spiritual care provider, social worker, or contact the hospice bereavement coordinator. Look forward, instead of always looking backward at the way things used to be. If you need help, ask. That's what your family, friends, and the hospice bereavement team are there for.

HOSPICE BEREAVEMENT SUPPORT

> *The friend who can be silent with us in a moment*
> *of despair or confusion; who can stay with us in an*
> *hour of grief and bereavement; who can tolerate not*
> *knowing, not curing, not healing and face with us*
> *the reality of our powerlessness, that is the friend*
> *who cares.*
>
> —**Henri Nouwen**, *Out of Solitude*

Hospice cares for the family long after a loved one's death. Although the Medicare hospice benefit promises bereavement support for up to one year, many hospices provide support for longer—for as long as needed.

When your loved one dies, the hospice care team may grieve too. They may attend the funeral or memorial service and share stories of your loved one. They may send a condolence card. Soon, however, the hospice care team will be replaced by the hospice bereavement team, which may consist of a spiritual care provider, a social worker, and volunteers. Their services usually begin shortly after the death. They will assess your ability to cope and will help in every way they can.

The hospice bereavement team might phone or visit. They might mail you literature, pamphlets, newsletters, and other materials related to grieving. They may provide bibliographies and educational booklets with information on coping with or grieving the loss of adults, teens, and children. Hospice may also have a lending library with books, pamphlets, videotapes, and audiotapes. They might host social events such as picnics and lunches, and they may hold a memorial service for loved ones who have died. They can also tell you about grief support groups in your area. You might use the Internet to find the best-selling books on grief and check them out of your public library.

In addition to information, support, and understanding, hospice may provide referrals to professionals who can help you work through your grief. If you need to talk to someone immediately, contact your hospice bereavement coordinator.

GETTING PAST THE PAIN

When we are grieving, we must identify all that has
been lost—and claim all that we still have.

—Steve Sims, hospice bereavement coordinator

Research suggests that bereaved individuals are more susceptible to illness, accidents, depression, and the development of destructive behaviors.

It is very important that you take care of yourself throughout the grieving process. Try to eat right, even if you aren't hungry. Try to get enough sleep, even if you are restless and dread the loneliness of your bed each night. Practice meditation and other relaxation techniques. Try to stay physically active and continue to challenge your mind. Attend to your own health care by regularly seeing your health practitioner.

Take care of yourself emotionally too. Don't dwell on regrets, on all the things you did or didn't do before your loved one died. Forgive yourself. Your loved one would forgive you. Make a list of all the things that you *did* do for your loved one. Know that you did all you could have done. If you have unfinished business with your loved one, you must cleanse the wound before it can heal. Talk aloud to your departed loved one. Write a letter, burn it, and scatter the ashes to the wind. Let it go.

Accept your grief. Feel it. Pay attention to today. Stay connected with friends and family. You might want to establish a new daily routine, one that includes exercising, calling friends, shopping, doing lunch, and the like. You will likely become friends with other bereaved people. Take it one day at a time, just as you did when caregiving. Live as your loved one would want you to live. As you work through your grief, learn to be a "creative survivor" by following these suggestions:

- Be consciously grateful for what you still have. Make a list.

- Write in a journal. Express your grief in words to help let it go.

- Let others know how you feel. "This is a sad day, a mad day, a blah day."

- Give other people room to be themselves. Encourage them to ask questions, talk, and cry if they feel like it.

- Make new friends by volunteering or joining a support group.

- Tell your story as often as you can. Listen to others share their stories too.

- When you find you are too preoccupied with grief, take a break from it. Rent a move, read a book, and so forth.

- Make a list of all the things that you *did* do for your loved one.

- Read books and articles or watch videos about grief.

- Get a pet. The warm, wet nose of a dog or the soothing purr of a cat can really help.

- Call your friends. Don't wait for them to call you—they may be afraid to call if they don't know quite what to say.

- Do something creative to honor your loved one.

- Ask yourself, "What have I learned from this experience?" Use what you have learned as your life continues.

Family and friends may offer lots of advice—take a vacation, get rid of your loved one's personal belongings, join a bridge club. Don't do something just because they suggest it. Do only what feels right.

BEREAVED CHILDREN

To children, the death of a parent can be a shattering experience. It may stun, shock, and frighten them. They may feel they are somehow responsible. They may also fear that their other parent will die, or that they themselves will die. Assure children that they are safe and loved. Let them know that it's okay to be sad or angry.

Listen. Be patient. Give children time to absorb what has happened. You might ask young children to picture a favorite toy in another room. They can see it in their mind and still love it without it being physically there. That is how they should think of their loved one now. Get them to talk. "What do you think happened?" "Why do you think that?" "How are you feeling?" With your help, children can come to understand the basic concepts of death—and they can begin to work through their grief.

Inform teachers and other adults about the death. This will save the child from having to make explanations and answer questions. It will also let adults understand the child's mood swings, allowing them to help the child deal with his or her emotions. Without such guidance, bereaved children may become aggressive, destructive, and uncooperative. Or, they may withdraw from everyone and everything.

Grieve together. In time, you and your children will feel less lonely and less afraid, and you will grow stronger.

Ten Suggestions to Help Children with Grief and Loss

1. As an adult, examine your own feelings around death and grief so you can talk with children as naturally as possible when opportunities arise.

2. Adults are children's role models. Be open with your feelings of grief and loss because children will mirror the adults in their lives.

3. Children will grieve differently based on developmental stage, personality and coping skills.

4. Offer honest, simple, and brief explanations.

5. Listen to and accept children's feelings and encourage healthy expression of those feelings.

6. Provide reassurance so children's basic needs will be met.

7. Maintain age-appropriate activities and interests because children often process their thoughts and feelings through play.

8. Encourage the use of expressive and creative arts such as drawing, painting, clay, music, and storytelling in order to work through feelings.

9. Rituals are a tool for recovery and an opportunity to memorialize a loved one. Encourage involvement and participation in events such as funerals, birthdays and anniversaries.

10. Remember that children will rework their grief at each developmental stage and gradually integrate the loss into their lives.

PRACTICAL MATTERS

The first few days after your loved one's death are full of activity: the funeral or memorial service, condolences from friends, phone calls, and the like. You are exhausted from the final days of care-giving and from saying goodbye. Nevertheless, there are practical matters that must be addressed.

If you need help, be sure to ask. Hopefully, most of the practical matters have been dealt with in advance. Even so, you will have a number of details to take care of. Do not sign any papers before reviewing them carefully. It never hurts to have someone you trust, such as an attorney, look over the papers too.

Gathering Important Documents

To claim benefits and tend to the estate, you will need several important documents—either copies or originals. If someone wants you to leave an original document with him or her for any reason, ask for a receipt.

The most important document is the death certificate. You will need the death certificate to transfer titles on vehicles, to change deeds to property, to file insurance claims, and to cancel credit cards, life insurance, mortgage payments, and medical policies. In addition, family members who fly home for the funeral may get a reduced airfare if they have a copy of the death certificate.

You can buy certified copies of this certificate through your funeral home or county health department, usually for a small fee.

Some agencies may accept uncertified copies of the death certificate, which could save you money. Always ask if a copy is sufficient. You may need a dozen or more death certificates, certified or not, depending on the complexity of your loved one's financial affairs. The death certificate is at the head of the list of important documents you will want to gather:

- Death certificate (both certified and uncertified copies).

- Marriage certificate (contact the county clerk where the wedding took place).

- Birth certificates of all dependent children (contact the county clerk where each child was born).

- Insurance policies.

- Social security numbers of your loved one and all survivors who might be eligible for benefits.

- Military service discharge papers.

- The will (original or copy).

- Deeds and titles to property.

- Loan and installment payment books and contracts.

- Stock certificates.

- Bank books (savings and checking).

- Last year's tax return.

- Vehicle registration.

- Outstanding debts.

If your loved one was in the military and you cannot find the discharge papers, you can write the Department of Defense at National Personnel Records Center, Military Personnel Records, 9700 Page Avenue, St. Louis, MO 63132, for a copy of the discharge.

Applying for Benefits

If your loved one was employed when she became ill, notify the employer to see if any insurance benefits, death benefits, profit sharing, or pension payments might be owed to you or the estate. You must also notify the Social Security Administration, insurance companies, unions, credit unions, and the like.

Former Employers

Unless your loved one was retired, check with former employers to see whether survivors are entitled to payments from a pension plan or life insurance policy. Also, employers can help determine if your loved one belonged to a union or professional organization that offers death benefits.

If your loved one was retired and receiving a pension, ask whether payments will be made to survivors at a reduced rate, or if they will cease entirely. If the illness was work-related, you may be entitled to workers' compensation benefits.

Social Security

Generally, a person is eligible for Social Security benefits if she has paid into Social Security for at least forty quarters. If your loved one had been receiving Social Security benefits, do not cash any checks that arrive after her death. These checks will need to be returned. If your loved one was not on Social Security, she may be eligible for two types of benefits.

Death benefit. A death benefit helps cover burial expenses. You can ask your funeral director to contact Social Security and have them apply the payment directly to the funeral bill. This payment is made only to eligible spouses or to children entitled to survivors' benefits.

Survivors' benefits. To be eligible for survivors' benefits, a spouse must be over age fifty-nine or caring for dependent children under age sixteen. Children may be eligible if they are under age eighteen or disabled. Check with your local Social Security office or call 1-800-772-1213.

If you are a spouse applying for Social Security benefits, you will need birth and death certificates of your loved one, your marriage certificate, birth certificates of any dependent children, Social

Security numbers for each of you, and a copy of your loved one's most recent federal income tax return.

Veterans' Benefits

If your loved one was a veteran, ask the funeral director to help you apply for veterans' benefits, or contact the Department of Veterans' Affairs (VA) by calling 1-800-827-1000. Benefits might include a lump-sum payment for burial expenses, an allowance toward a cemetery plot, and a headstone or grave marker at no charge. Burial in a national cemetery is free to a veteran, her spouse, and dependent children. If your loved one was receiving disability benefits from the VA, you and your children might be entitled to monthly payments of some kind.

Insurance Policies

Check all life and casualty insurance policies for benefits. Your loved one might also have mortgage insurance, loan insurance, and credit card insurance. If your loved one had insurance through a credit union, trade union, or fraternal organization, one of these organizations may provide survivors' benefits or cover part of the burial expenses.

Usually, proceeds from insurance policies are paid directly to the named beneficiary. It is important to file claims as soon as possible, especially if you are concerned about your finances. You might have an option between taking a lump-sum or receiving payments over a number of months or years. A financial advisor can help you decide which option is best for you.

Credit Cards and Installment Payments

To protect your credit rating, make credit card payments on time. Cancel any credit cards issued solely in your loved one's name. For jointly held accounts, notify each company of your loved one's death and ask them to remove her name from the account. Some credit card companies will cancel debt upon the death of a cardholder, so be sure to ask. Also ask if your loved one had credit card insurance. Review all other debts and installment payments to determine whethr any will cancel the debt.

Updating Insurance Policies, Bank Accounts, and Titles

After your loved one's death, you may need to change your insurance policies. For example, if you have life insurance and your loved one was the beneficiary, you must now name a new beneficiary. If you have medical insurance through your loved one's employer, you and your dependent children may continue coverage for up to thirty-six months—if you pay the premiums—under a federal law called COBRA. Eventually, you will need to apply for new medical insurance. Homeowners' and automobile insurance policies will also need to be updated.

You must change the title on all vehicles owned by the deceased. Contact your state department of motor vehicles to learn how.

Any joint bank accounts that you and your loved one shared will automatically pass to you. However, you should see a bank representative to change the title and signature cards on the account. Jointly held stocks or bonds will also pass to you, but again, the titles should be changed. If the stocks and bonds were held in your loved one's name, they will need to go through probate.

In most states, you are permitted to access a jointly held safe deposit box. However, if the safe deposit box was held in your loved one's name, only the will (and any other materials related to the death) can be removed before the will has been probated.

If you have your own will, and it states that property should pass to your loved one upon your death, you will need to update your will.

Executing the Will

If your loved one had a will, it may be in a safe deposit box, in a family safe, or with your family lawyer. The will details how your loved one wants her property and possessions to be distributed.

If a person dies without a will, that person is said to have died *intestate*. In this case, property and possessions are distributed according to state law—typically, first to a surviving spouse, then to children, and then to other blood relatives. Or a spouse may receive half the estate while the children divide the other half. (This is referred to as passing possessions on to the next of kin.)

Insurance proceeds, Series E bonds, death benefits (such as social security or VA benefits), and jointly owned property and bank accounts will bypass the will and go directly to the designated beneficiary or joint owner. The rest of the estate may need to go through probate.

Trusts

A trust is a legal arrangement in which a person or financial institution (the trustee) manages assets for the benefit of someone else (the beneficiary). The person who creates and funds the trust, in your case your loved one, is called the "grantor."

The grantor creates a trust in her will, to take effect upon her death. Or the grantor can create a "living trust," providing funds to be used for the grantor if she is alive but incapacitated.

Trusts can be either revocable or irrevocable. As the terms imply, a revocable trust can be changed or terminated at any time. An irrevocable trust, on the other hand, cannot be changed or terminated after it is signed. Usually, a revocable trust is preferred.

Probate

Probate is a legal process to open and close an estate. It documents legal ownership of inherited property. The purpose is to pay a deceased person's debts and distribute the estate to the rightful heirs.

To file for probate, take the will and a copy of the death certificate to your local probate court. A judge will determine if the will is valid. The will may name a *personal representative* or *executor* of the estate. Most courts will honor this decision. If there is no will, the court will appoint an executor.

The executor must file a petition with the court after the death. Once a petition is filed, the court issues a letter stating that this individual accepts responsibility for collecting assets, paying debts, and distributing the remaining assets. The personal representative usually opens a bank account in the name of the deceased person's estate, collects payments, sells property, and pays bills. After probate is completed, the personal representative distributes assets to the heirs as directed by the will or the court.

Because probate is often complex, it may be expensive and

time-consuming. You may need a lawyer. Even with a will, an estate will need to go through probate if it involves sole ownership of real estate or stocks and bonds.

Paying Taxes

Federal estate tax. A federal estate tax may need to be paid before the estate is distributed. Currently, estate tax is due only on estates that exceed an applicable exclusion amount. For 2008, the applicable exclusion amount is $2,000,000. In the future the exclusion amount will increase, so it would be advisable to consult the Internal Revenue Service Web site, www.irs.gov or a tax lawyer.

Inheritance tax. Some states charge no inheritance tax; others charge 1 percent or more. Generally, any estate that pays a federal estate tax must file a state estate tax return. Check with your state tax department. Because state and federal tax laws are complicated and constantly changing, you may wish to consult a tax professional for information on current tax laws.

Income tax. Your loved one's federal and state income taxes are due for the year of her death. If there are dependent children and the surviving spouse did not remarry, the spouse can file jointly for the year of death and for two additional years.

Other Financial Matters

If your loved one had debts, the executor will generally pay these debts from the estate account. However, to continue or establish your own credit rating, if you have shared debts, such as mortgage payments and utility bills, you should continue to pay them.

If you find yourself in financial difficulty after the death of your loved one, you can apply for emergency funds from your local social services department. This is not a good time to make important financial decisions, such as whether to sell your house. Give yourself time to sort things out.

MOVING ON

But if grief is resolved, why do we still feel a sense of loss come anniversaries and holidays, and even when we least expect it? Why do we feel a lump in the throat, even six years after the loss? It is because healing does not mean forgetting, and because moving on with life does not mean that we don't take a part of our lost loved one with us.

—Adolfo Quezada, "By Choosing to Confront Grief, We Can Overcome Our Loss"

It will never be all right that your loved one has died. You must accept it and move on, just as you did when you first learned of the terminal illness. Working through your grief does not mean forgetting your loved one. It simply means that you can live your life fully in spite of your loss. You may even grow as you begin to experience a "new normal" for your life.

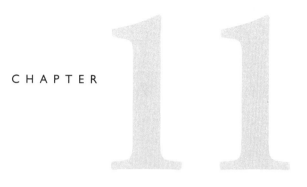

Resources: Where to Find Information and Help

A great deal of information and assistance is available to hospice patients and their families. Several books on hospice, home care, death and dying, and grief are available at your local library. In addition, many organizations can provide referrals and other information. You can find further resources on the Internet. Your hospice team may also be able to suggest additional resources.

BOOKS AND PAMPHLETS

Information about Hospice

All About Hospice: A Consumer's Guide. Washington, DC: Foundation for Hospice and Homecare, 1991.

Beresford, Larry. *The Hospice Handbook: A Complete Guide.* New York: Little, Brown and Company, 1993.

Lattanzi-Licht, Marcia, John J. Mahoney and Galen W. Miller. *The Hospice Choice: In Pursuit of a Peaceful Death.* New York: Fireside, 1998.

Munley, Anne. *The Hospice Alternative: A New Context for Death and Dying.* New York: Basic Books, 1986.

Stoddard, Sandol. *The Hospice Movement: A Better Way of Caring for the Dying.* London: Vintage Books, 1992.

Information about Home Care

American Dietetic Association. *The American Dietetic Association's Complete Food and Nutrition Guide.* New York: Wiley, 2002.

Arras, John D., ed. *Bringing the Hospital Home: Ethical and Social Implications of High-Tech Home Care.* Baltimore: Johns Hopkins University Press, 1995.

Berman, Claire. *Caring for Yourself While Caring for Your Aging Parents.* New York: Henry Holt and Company, 2005.

Bintliff, Shay. "Caregiving for Caregivers." *The Brown University Long-Term Care Quality Advisor.* July 1998.

Carter, Rosalynn. *Helping Yourself Help Others: A Book for Caregivers.* New York: Three Rivers Press, 1995.

Duda, Deborah. *Coming Home: A Guide to Home Care for the Terminally Ill.* Santa Fe, NM.: Aurora Press, 1984.

Fairview Pain and Palliative Care Center. *When Your Pain Flares Up: Easy, Proven Techniques for Managing Chronic Pain.* Minneapolis, Fairview Press, 2002.

Karnes, Barbara. "A Time to Live: Living with a Life-Threatening Illness." P.O. Box 335, Stilwell, KS 66085. 1996.

Little, Deborah Whiting. *Home Care for the Dying: A Reassuring, Comprehensive Guide to Physical and Emotional Care.* Jackson, TN: Main Street Publications, 1985.

McCann, Robert M., et al. "Comfort Care for Terminally Ill Patients." *Journal of the American Medical Association* 272 (1994): 1263–1266.

McFarlane, Rodger. *The Complete Bedside Companion.* New York: Fireside, 1999.

Miller, James E. *The Caregiver's Book: Caring for Another, Caring for Yourself.* Minneapolis: Augsburg Fortress, 1996.

Sankar, Andrea. *Dying at Home: A Family Guide for Caregiving.* Baltimore: Johns Hopkins University Press, 2000.

Weihofen, Donna. *The Cancer Survival Cookbook.* Hoboken, NJ: John Wiley & Sons, 2002.

Wilkinson, James A. *A Family Caregiver's Guide to Planning and Decision Making for the Elderly.* Minneapolis: Fairview Press, 1999.

Information about Death, Dying, and Grief

Amatuzio, Janis. *Forever Ours: Real Stories of Immortality and Living from a Forensic Pathologist.* Novato CA: New World Library, 2007.

Babcock, Elise. *When Life Becomes Precious.* New York: Bantam Books, 1997.

Bloomfield, Harold H., Melba Colgrove, and Peter McWilliams. *How to Survive the Loss of a Love.* Allen Park, MI: Mary Books/Prelude Press, 2004.

Boss, Pauline. *Ambiguous Loss: Learning to Live with Grief.* Cambridge, MA: Harvard U Press, 2000.

Brookes, Tim. *Signs of Life: A Memoir of Dying and Discovery.* Hinesburg, VT: Upper Access, 2000.

Byock, Ira. *Dying Well: Peace and Possibilities at the End of Life.* New York: Riverhead Books, 1998.

————. *Dying Well: The Prospect for Growth at the End of Life.* New York: Riverhead Books, 1997.

Callanan, Maggie. *Final Gifts: Understanding the Special Awareness, Needs, and Communications of the Dying.* New York: Bantam Books, 1997.

Doka, Kenneth J., ed. *Living with Grief: At Work, at School, at Worship.* Levittown, PA: Brunner/Mazel, 1999.

Edelman, Hope. *Motherless Daughters: The Legacy of Loss.* 2nd edition. Cambridge, MA: Da Capo Press, 2006

Fairview Health Services. *Caring for a Loved One at the End of Life: At Home or with Hospice Care.* Minneapolis: Fairview Press, 2006.

Fairview Health Services. *Journey through the Dying Process: When a Loved One Is in the Hospital or Another Medical Setting.* Minneapolis: Fairview Press, 2006.

James, John W.; Russell Friedman. *Grief Recovery Handbook: The Action Program for Moving Beyond Death, Divorce, and Other Losses.* New York: HarperPerennial, 1998.

Karnes, Barbara. "Gone from My Sight: The Dying Experience." P.O. Box 335, Stilwell, Kansas 66085. 1986.

———. "My Friend, I Care: The Grief Experience." P.O. Box 335, Stilwell, KS 66085. 1991.

Kübler-Ross, Elisabeth. *On Death and Dying.* New York: Scribner, 1997.

——— and David Kessler. *On Grief and Grieving: Finding the meaning of grief through the five stages of loss.* New York: Scribner, 2007.

Levang, Elizabeth. *Remembering with Love: Messages of Hope for the First Year of Grieving and Beyond.* Minneapolis: Fairview Press, 1996.

———. *When Men Grieve: Why Men Grieve Differently and How You Can Help.* Minnneapolis: Fairview Presss, 1998.

Levy, Alexander. *Orphaned Adults: Understanding and Coping with Grief and Change after the Death of Our Parents.*

Lynch, Gayle. *In Sickness and in Health: One Woman's Story of Love, Loss, and Healing.* Minneapolis: Fairview Press, 2006.

Morrison, R. Sean, and Jane Morris. "When There Is No Cure." *Geriatrics.* July 1995.

Nuland, Sherwin B. *How We Die: Reflections on Life's Final Chapter.* New York: Vintage Books, 1995.

Quill, Timothy E. *Death and Dignity: Making Choices and Taking Charge.* New York: W. W. Norton and Company, 1994.

Samples, Pat. *Daily Comforts for Caregivers.* Minneapolis, Fairview Press, 1999.

Tobin, Daniel R. *Peaceful Dying: The Step-by-Step Guide to Preserving Your Dignity, Your Choice, and Your Inner Peace at the End of Life.* Reading, Mass.: Perseus Books, 1998.

Wass, Hannelore, ed. *Dying: Facing the Facts.* 3rd ed. London: Taylor & Francis, 1995.

Westberg, Granger E. *Good Grief: A Constructive Approach to the Problem of Loss.* Philadelphia, PA: Fortress Press, 1997.

Whitmore Hickman, Martha. *Healing After Loss: Daily Meditations for Working Through Grief.* New York: Avon Books, 1994.

Winters, Paul A., ed. *Death and Dying: Opposing Viewpoints.* San Diego: Greenhaven Press, 1997.

Zonnebelt-Smeenge, Susan and Robert C. DeVries. *Getting to the Other Side of Grief: Overcoming the Loss of a Spouse.* Grand Rapids, MI: Baker Books, 1998.

Information about Legal and Financial Matters

"Funeral and Burial; Wills and Living Trusts," Washington, DC: AARP. www.aarp.org. 1999.

Medicare: Hospice Benefits. Washington, D.C.: U.S. Department of Health and Human Services Health Care Financing Administration. Publication No. HCFA 02154, 1994.

Wilkinson, James A. *A Family Caregiver's Guide to Planning and Decision Making for the Elderly.* Minneapolis: Fairview Press, 1999.

Information about Children's Grief

Fairview Health Services. *A Teen's Guide to Coping: When a Loved One Is Sick and Preparing to Die.* Minneapolis: Fairview Press, 2006.

Fairview Health Services. *Helping Kids Cope: When a Loved One Is Sick and Preparing to Die.* Minneapolis: Fairview Press, 2006.

Fine, Judylaine. *Afraid to Ask: A Book for Families to Share about Cancer.* New York: Harper Trophey, 1986.

Gravelle, Karen. *Teenagers Face to Face with Bereavement.* Lincoln, NE: iUniverse, 2000.

Grollman, Earl A. *Talking about Death: A Dialogue Between Parent and Child.* Boston: Beacon Press, 1991.

Heegaard, Marge. *When Someone Has a Very Serious Illness: Children Can Learn to Cope with Loss and Change.* Minneapolis: Woodland Press, 1992.

———. *When Someone Very Special Dies: Children Can Learn to Cope with Grief.* Minneapolis: Woodland Press, 1988.

Huntley, Theresa. *Helping Children Grieve.* Minneapolis: Augsburg Fortress, 2002.

Latour, Kathy. *For Those Who Live: Helping Children Cope with the Death of a Brother or Sister.* Omaha, NE: Centering Corporation, 1987.

Le Shan, Eda J. *Learning to Say Goodbye: When a Parent Dies.* Madison, WI: Demco Media, 1988.

Libby, Larry. *Someday Heaven.* Grand Rapids, MI: Zonderkidz, 2001.

Miles, Miska. *Annie and the Old One.* Boston: Little, Brown and Company, 1985.

Rando, Therese A. *How to Go On Living When Someone You Love Dies.* New York: Bantam Books, 1991.

Schwiebert, Pat et al. *A Recipe for Healing after Loss.* Portland, OR: Grief Watch, 1999.

Silverman, Janis. *Help Me Say Goodbye: Activities for Helping Kids Cope When a Special Person Dies.* Minneapolis: Fairview Press, 1999.

Turner, Mary. *Talking with Young Children about Death.* Philadelphia: Jessica Kingsley Publishers, 1998.

Zimmermann, Susan. *Writing to Heal the Soul: Transforming Grief and Loss Through Writing.* New York: Three Rivers Press, 2002.

ORGANIZATIONS AND AGENCIES

AIDS and HIV

Center for Disease Control National AIDS Hotline
CDC-INFO
1-800-CDC-INFO (232-4636)(24 hours)
www.cdc.gov/hiv

Information, referral services, and publications about HIV and AIDS.

National AIDS Fund
729 15th Street NW, 9th Floor
Washington, DC 20005
1-888-234-2437
www.aidsfund.org

National Association of People with AIDS
8401 Colesville Road, Suite 750
Silver Spring, MD 2010
(240) 247-0880
www.napwa.org

Information and referrals.

Alzheimer's Disease

Alzheimer's Association
225 N. Michigan Avenue, Floor 17
Chicago, IL 60601
1-800-272-3900
www.alz.org

Referrals to over 200 local chapters nationwide.

Cancers and Tumors

American Brain Tumor Association
2720 River Road, Suite 146
Des Plaines, IL 60018
1-800-886-2282
www.abta.org

Provides publications on various levels and types of tumors, a support
group listing, a newsletter, and a pen-pal program. Social workers are
also on staff.

American Cancer Society
National Office
1599 Clifton Road N.E.
Atlanta, GA 30329-4251
1-800-ACS-2345
www.cancer.org

Call for the number for your local division. Most local divisions can provide current information on cancer treatments, financial assistance, local
resources, and local support groups. They may also help arrange for walk-
ers, wheelchairs, hospital beds, and other medical equipment at no cost.

American Lung Association
61 Broadway, 6th Floor
New York, NY 10006
1-800-548-8252
(212) 315-8700
www.lungusa.org

Offers publications and conducts educational programs.

Bloch Cancer Foundation, Inc.
One H&R Block Way
Kansas City, MO 64111-1812
1-800-433-0464
www.blochcancer.org

Volunteer organization offers resources, peer counseling, and
support groups.

Bone Marrow Transplant Family Support Network
20411 W. 12 Mile Rd.,Suite 108
Southfield, MI 48076
1-800-LINK-BMT
(800-546-5268)
248-358-1886
www.nbmtlink.org/resources_support/sc/sc_resource.htm

National network for patients and families.

CanCare
9575 Katy Freeway, Suite 428
Houston, TX 77024
(713) 461-0028
www.cancare.org

Church-based, volunteer ministry offering support for cancer patients
and family. Provides a newsletter and referrals.

Cancer Care, Inc.
275 7th Avenue
New York, NY 10001
1-800-813-HOPE (4673)
www.CancerCare.org

Free individual and group telephone counseling, worksite
programs, and referrals.

Cancer Counseling, Inc.
4101 Greenbriar, Suite 317
Houston, TX 77098
(713) 520-9873
www.cancercounseling.info

Offers free professional counseling and educational programs,
numerous educational materials, and a newsletter.

Cancer Hope Network
Two North Road, Suite A
Chester, NJ 07930
1-877-HOPENET (467-3638)
(908) 233-1130
www.cancerhopenetwork.org

Matches volunteers with similar types of cancer to provide support
by phone or in person. Also publishes a newsletter.

Candlelighters Childhood Cancer Foundation
PO Box 498
Kensignton, MD 20895-0498
1-800-366-2223
www.candlelighters.org
staff@candlelighters.org

Support services for families of children with cancer.

Children's Leukemia Research Association, Inc.
585 Stewart Avenue, Suite 18
Garden City, NY 11530
(516)-222-1944
www.childrensleukemia.org

Free brochures and newsletters.

Coping Magazine—Coping with Cancer
P.O. Box 682268
Franklin, TN 37068-2268
(615) 790-2400
www.copingmag.com

National cancer magazine for patients and caregivers.

International Myeloma Foundation
12650 Riverside Drive
Suite 206
North Hollywood, CA 91607
1-800-452-CURE (2873)
www.myeloma.org
PheIMF@myeloma.org

Provides brochures, a quarterly newsletter, patient and family seminars, scientific workshops, and research grants.

Leukemia Society of America
1311 Mamaroneck Avenue
White Plains, NY 10605
1-800-955-4572
www.leukemia.org

Brochures, referrals, and support groups.

Lymphoma Research Foundation of America, Inc.
8800 Venice Boulevard, Suite 207
Los Angeles, CA 90034
Helpline: 1-800-500-9976
www.lymphoma.org
Email: *lrfa@aol.com*

Educational materials and a newsletter.

Memorial Sloan-Kettering Cancer Center
Post-Treatment Resource Program
1275 York Avenue
New York, NY 10021
(212) 212-639-2000
800-525-2225
www.mskcc.org

Cancer research, support group for cancer survivors.

National Brain Tumor Foundation
22 Battery Street, Suite 612
San Francisco, CA 94111-5520
1-800-934-CURE (2873)
www.braintumor.org

Raises funds to support patients and their families.

National Cancer Institute
Cancer Information Center
6116 Executive Boulevard
Room 3036A
Bethesda, MD 20892
1-800-422-6237
(301) 402-5874
www.cancer.gov

Nationwide information service offering several free brochures.

Caregiving

AARP
601 E Street N.W.
Washington, DC 20049
1-888-687-2277
www.aarp.org

Free informational pamphlets include "The Caregiver Resource Kit" and "Information on Home Care Services."

U.S. Administration on Aging
U.S. Health and Human Services
1 Massachusetts Avenue
Washington, DC 20201
(202) 619-0724
www.*aoa.gov*

Aging Network Services
4400 East-West Highway, Suite 907
Bethesda, MD 20814
(301) 657-4329
www.*agingnets.com*

Aging with Dignity
P.O. Box 1661
Tallahassee, FL 32302-1661
1-888-594-7437
www.agingwithdignity.org; fivewishes@aol.com

Provides the "Five Wishes" document, which includes living wills and healthcare proxy choices for thirty-three states.

Anderson Network
1515 Holcombe Boulevard, Box 216
Houston, TX 77030
1-800-345-6324 (support line)
(713) 792-2553
www.mdanderson.org/departments/andersonnet

Volunteers offer support to cancer patients and their families through a national telephone network. Also provide a newsletter, an annual conference for patients and caregivers, and a quality of life program.

Children of Aging Parents
P.O. Box 167
Richboro, PA 18954
1-800-227-7294
www.caps4caregivers.org

Eldercare Locator
927 15th Street N.W., 6th Floor
Washington, DC 20005
1-800-677-1116
www.eldercare.gov

National Family Caregivers Association
10400 Connecticut Avenue, Suite 500
Kensington, MD 20895-3944
1-800-896-3650
www.nfcacares.org

Provides a resource guide and a newsletter on caregiving.

Death

Association for Death Education and Counseling
National Office
60 Revere Drive, Suite 500
Northbrook IL 60062
www.adec.org
847-509-0403

Candlelighters Childhood Cancer Foundation
P.O. Box 498
Kensington, MD 20895
1-800-366-2223
www.candlelighters.org
staff@candlelighters.org

Support services for families of children with cancer.

Growth House, Inc.
415-863-3045
www.growthhouse.org

Resources on end-of-life issues such as hospice and home care, palliative care, pain management, death with dignity, and bereavement.

Project on Death in America
Open Society Institute
400 W. 59th Street
New York, NY 10019
212-548-0600
www.soros.org/death/index.htm

Seeks to understand and transform the forces that have created and sustained our current culture of dying.

Financial and Legal Matters

Aging with Dignity
P.O. Box 1661
Tallahassee, FL 32302-1661
1-800-562-1931
(850) 681-2010
www.agingwithdignity.org
fivewishes@aol.com

Provides the "Five Wishes" document, which includes living wills and healthcare proxy choices for thirty-three states.

Concern for Dying—An Educational Council
250 West 57th Street
New York, NY 10107

Concerned primarily with living wills, death with dignity, and other patients' rights.

U.S. Department of Health and Human Services
Centers for Medicare and Medical Services
7500 Security Boulevard
Baltimore, MD 21244-1850
1-800-772-1213
www.cms.hhs.gov

U.S. Department of Veterans Affairs (VA) Office
1-800-827-1000,
www.va.gov

VA Benefits, local or nationwide.

Internal Revenue Service
(See the government section in your phone book.)
Form #448 "A Guide to Federal Estate and Gift Taxation"
Form #559 "Tax Information for Survivors, Executors, and
Administrators"
Form #706 "Federal Estate Taxes"
www.irs.gov

National Personnel Records Center
Military Personnel
Records"
9700 Page Avenue
St. Louis, MO 63132
314-801-0800
www.archives.gov/st-louis/military-personnel
mprstatus@nara.gov

Funeral Planning

Funeral Consumers Alliance
33 Patchen Road
South Burlington, VT 05403
1-800-765-0107
www.funerals.org

Information on planning inexpensive funerals.

National Funeral Directors Association
13625 Bishops Drive
Brookfield, WI 53005
1-800-228-6332
www.nfda.org

Organization of licensed funeral directors and embalmers.

Grief

The Accord
1930 Bishop Lane, Suite 947
Louisville, KY 40218
(502) 458-0260

Enclose a $3 check for this publication "Holiday Help: Coping for the Bereaved."

The Beginning Experience
1657 Commerce Drive
South Bend, IN 46628
1(574)283-0279
1-866-610-8877
www.beginningexperience.org

Peer ministry for separated and divorced women.

Bereavement Publications, Inc.
P.O. Box 61
Montrose, CO 81402
1-888-604-4673
www.breavementmag.com

Offers the publication "Living with Loss: Hope and Healing for the Body, Mind, and Spirit."

Grief and Loss
AARP
1601 E Street N.W.
Washington, DC 20049
(202) 434-2260
www.aarp.org/griefandloss

Referrals to local grief support services, publications, books on widowhood.

Grief Recovery Institute

P.O. Box 6061-382
Sherman Oaks, CA 91413
1-818-907-9600
www.grief-recovery.com

THEOS Foundation (They Help Each Other Spiritually)
322 Boulevard of the Allies, Suite 105
Pittsburgh, PA 15222-1919
(412) 471-7770

For widows and widowers. Information and referral to local chapters.
Enclose a self-addressed, stamped envelope for their publication, "Grief
Is Not a Weakness."

Heart Disease

American Heart Association
7272 Greenville Avenue
Dallas, TX 75231
1-800-AHA-USA1
www.americanheart.org

Committed to reducing disability and death from cardiovascular
disease and stroke.

Hospice

American Academy of Hospice and Palliative Medicine
4700 W. Lake Avenue
Glenview, IL 60025
(847) 375-4712
www.aahpm.org

American Hospice Foundation
2120 L Street N.W., Suite 200
Washington, DC 20037
(202) 223-0204
www.americanhospice.org

Children's Hospice International
1101 King Street, Suite 360
Alexandria, VA 22314
1-800-24CHILD
(703) 684-0330
www.chionline.org

Resource and administration for children's hospice programs.

Fairview Hospice
2450 26th Avenue S.
Minneapolis, MN 55406
(612) 672-2600
www.fairview.org/hospice

Hospicelink
1-800-331-1620

Up-to-date directory of hospice and palliative care programs throughout the United States.

Hospice Foundation of America
1621 Connecticut Avenue N.W., Suite 300
Washington, DC 20009
1-800-854-3402
www.hospicefoundation.org

International Association for Hospice and Palliative Care
5535 Memorial Drive, Suite F
(936) 321-9846
866-374-2472
Houston, TX 77007
www.hospicecare.com/

National Hospice & Palliative Care Organization (NHPCO)
1700 Diagonal Road, Suite 625
Alexandria, VA 22314
(703) 837-1500
1-800-658-8898
www.nho.org

A nonprofit organization devoted to increasing awareness of and access
to hospice care through the financial support of education and research.

Living Wills and Advanced Directives

Aging with Dignity
P.O. Box 1661
Tallahassee, FL 32302-1661
1-800-594-7437
(850) 681-2010
www.agingwithdignity.org
fivewishes@aol.com

Provides the "Five Wishes" document, which includes living wills and healthcare proxy choices for thirty-three states.

Compassion & Choices
P.O. Box 101810
Denver, CO 80250
1-800-247-7421
www.compassionandchoices.org

Provides information on living wills and medical powers of attorney.

Lung Disease

American Lung Association
61 Broadway, 6th Floor
New York, NY 10006
1-800-586-4872
(212) 315-8700
www.lungusa.org

Offers publications and conducts educational programs.

Medicare

AARP
601 E Street N.W.
Washington, DC 20049
1-888-687-2277
www.aarp.org

Offers a free booklet, "Information on Medicare and Health Insurance for Older People."

Medicare Hotline
1-800-633-4227

Call for a free copy of "The Medicare Handbook."

National Hospice & Palliative Care Organization (NHPCO)
1700 Diagonal Road, Suite 625
Alexandria, VA 22314
(703) 837-1500
1-800-658-8898
www.nho.org

Offers a booklet titled "Hospice Under Medicare."

Multiple Sclerosis

Multiple Sclerosis Association of America
706 Haddonfield Road
Cherry Hill, NJ 08002
1-800-532-7667
www.msaa.com

Pain

American Chronic Pain Association
P.O. Box 850
Rocklin, CA 95677
(916) 632-0922
1-800-533-3231
www.theacpa.org

Provides a support system, guidelines for selecting a pain management unit, and referrals to over 600 chapters.

Memorial Sloan-Kettering Cancer Center
1275 York Avenue
New York, NY 10065
888-675-7722
www.mskcc.org/mskcc/html/474.cfm

For information on managing cancer pain.

National Chronic Pain Outreach Association
P.O. Box 274
Millboro, VA 24460
540-862-9437
www.chronicpain.org

An information clearinghouse with publications and referrals to pain clinics, pain management specialists, and pain support groups. Publishes brochures and a quarterly newsletter, *Lifeline*, which offers practical techniques for coping with pain.

Urologic Disease

American Urologic Association Foundation
1000 Corporate Boulevard
Linthicum, MO 21090
866-746-4282
(410) 689-3700
www.auafoundation.org
ww.urologyhealth.org

Provides free literature on prostate cancer.

Index